GUIDE
TO
HOMOEOPATHY

GUIDE TO HOMOEOPATHY

Martin Coventry

CAXTON REFERENCE

CONTENTS

This book is a concise guide to homoeopathy and the remedies used to treat symptoms of illness. Homoeopathy is a complementary therapy which works along with traditional medicine. Many illnesses require a precise medical diagnosis and may require urgent help from the medical services – homoeopathy by itself is not suitable for all conditions.

The first part of the book describes the history and methodology of homoeopathy, which was founded by Dr Samuel Hahnemann at the beginning of the 19th century. Information is supplied on how remedies work, how they are prepared, and how they should be administered.

The second part of the book is an A to Z gazetteer of a selection of homoeopathic remedies, describing over 200 remedies. Each entry begins with the name of the remedy and alternative names, while the next part describes the symptom picture. Additional information includes things which improve or exacerbate symptoms, constitutional types, derivation and preparation of remedy, and background.

The third part lists details of some common ailments and conditions. An index of symptoms concludes the book.

History

The word homoeopathy is from the Greek *homoeos* meaning similar or the same and pathos meaning feeling or suffering. It is based on the concept that 'like cures like'. The closer the match between the symptoms caused by a disease or condition to the remedy picture – the symptoms the remedy causes in normal, healthy individuals – the better the therapeutic effect.

Homoeopathy was developed by Dr Samuel Hahnemann, a German physician and chemist at the beginning of the 19th century. Hahnemann believed that the medical treatments of his time often made patients worse, rather than helping them. Many treatments involved widespread use of potentially toxic substances such as mercury. Indeed, he believed that the whole basis of conventional medicine was flawed, that it was not necessarily beneficial to treat a symptom with a remedy which had an opposite effect in an attempt to suppress or remove that symptom.

Hahnemann had noticed that quinine from cinchona bark, a treatment for malaria, could produce symptoms of malaria when taken in small doses by a healthy person (he tested this on himself – he used himself, family, friends and students to prove many substances). Between 1790 and 1810 he carried out a series of experiments, numerous trials called 'provings', which showed that substances induce standard signs and symptoms when taken by normal, healthy people. He decided that symptoms of illness where actually the body's method of combating that illness. His theory was that small doses of herbs and compounds which produced symptoms of an illness could then be used to treat that illness. In other words, the medicine whose symptom picture most closely resembled the disease or condition was the one which is most likely to result in a cure. This was an ancient philosophy, which was proposed by Hippocrates in the 5th century, but had largely gone out of favour. The ethical oath taken by new doctors in orthodox medicine is named after Hippocrates.

Hanhemann's theories said that the outward physical signs of an illness represented the body's best attempt to heal itself. He used the term homoeopathy to describe his system of using treatments and medicines which imitated the illness in some way, rather than the more usual method of treating symptoms with a stronger opponent in an attempt to remove or reduce symptoms. He also recommended a good diet and clean and sanitary living conditions as a means of maintaining health and reducing the chances of becoming ill. Many of the substances he proposed as cures, however. were extremely poisonous in larger doses, and potentially fatal.

Although the early Greek physicians had used similars to some treatments, Hahnemann developed a systematic philosophy and methodology for diagnosis and treatment. His approach was never accepted by more orthodox medical practitioners and he was ridiculed by many. In 1831, however, there was a cholera epidemic in central Europe, and Hahnemann recommended using camphor, which cured many of the sick. When Hahnemann died, he left important technical manuals, and homoeopaths were training and practising throughout Europe and America. One of those cured in the cholera epidemic in 1831 was Dr Frederick Quin, an English medical practitioner, who went on to found a homoeopathic hospital in London in 1849. Camphor was used in another cholera epidemic in Britain, and again proved its worth.

Homoeopathy was well established in the United States of America, and was further researched and improved by practitioners such as Dr Constantine Hering and Dr James Tyler Kent. Hering invented the 'laws of cure', which formulated the idea that symptoms moved from one part of the body to another as treatment progressed. Kent introduced the idea of constitutional types, which is now the basis of homoeopathy, which takes into account the physical and emotional make-up of the person as well as symptoms of illness.

In the late 19th century further work was undertaken by Wilhelm Heinrich Schussler, a German homoeopath. Schussler moved away from a holistic approach and proposed that many conditions and symptoms were caused by deficiency in tiny quantities of minerals or tissue salts, which could then be replaced. Schussler proposed there were twelve such essential salts.

Interest in homoeopathy waned in the first few decades of the 20th century as a split developed in homoeopathic practice, but interest has grown again towards the end of the century.

Materia Medica

The system, which lists detailed information about all homoeopathic remedies including their source, is based on treating the sick person rather than a set of rules about illnesses and diseases. As mentioned above, in 1790 Hahnemann was carrying out some tests using cinchona, Peruvian bark, and ingested some himself. He felt numb, cold and drowsy. He also experienced anxiety and palpitations. The symptoms were similar to ague or intermittent fever, now known to be a form of malaria, which was one of the diseases that Peruvian bark was prescribed for. Over the next twenty years he administered medical substances to healthy people, himself or his students, and recorded the symptoms that they induced. This enabled Hahnemann to build up a list of symptoms caused by these remedies.

At the moment the list of homoeopathic treatments includes over 2,000 remedies, of which over 200 are described in the following pages. Most of the treatments are vegetable in origin: flowers, fruits, seeds, nuts, bark, leaves, rhizome, roots. Many can be extremely poisonous and even deadly; others are quite common, well-accepted medicinal plants or herbs which continue to be used in herbal or orthodox medicine to this day.

Other treatments are mineral and include metals, salts, alkalis and acids, while some are animal in origin and include the poisons of snakes, spiders, and toads; as well as bodily secretions, milk, tissue extracts and also some disease tissue such as abscesses or syphilis, which are known as 'nosodes'.

Hahnemann had proposed that many people had a chronic constitutional weakness which was the result of an underlying disease which had come a previous generation of the person's family. This concept was called 'miasm', from the Greek word for pollution, and he believed that this weakness meant that some people were never truly healthy and would always have symptoms of the illness. Hahnemann identified three main miasms: psora from scabies, sycosis from gonorrhoea, and syphilinum from syphilis.

This latter idea was further investigated by Wilhelm Lux amid considerable controversy – the idea being that the remedy, the 'nosode', was actually prepared from diseased tissue itself that the remedy was to cure. Examples of substances he investigated are Medorrhinum (from gonorrhoea) and Tuberculinium. Other miasms have since been identified, although there is now a more modern interpretation of this theory.

There is no danger, however, from these remedies: they are so diluted that none of the original tissue ends up in the remedy.

Principles

Homoeopathy is also based on the philosophy of holistic natural healing, which is based not just on curing disease but maintaining a healthy lifestyle. Illness is a disturbance of the vital force and results in physical, mental and emotional symptoms which are unique to each person. Therefore it is important that all symptoms are considered before starting any treatment. The patient's lifestyle, emotional well-being and feelings are assessed as well as physical symptoms. Their appearance, build, hair colour and other physical characteristics are also noted.

The method of treatment involves one particular remedy for the whole patient which is based on an assessment of the totality of symptoms matched with various remedies until the closest match is found. The power and effect of the treatments are related to the response of individual patients. If more than one remedy is administered at a time then it is difficult to know which one has worked.

As the principle of the treatment is based on stimulating a self-healing process rather than correcting an abnormality large or prolonged doses are unnecessary and may also be ineffectual. Besides which large doses of the some of the remedy ingredients would be extremely harmful. The smallest possible dose is used and treatment is only repeated if absolutely necessary. The remedy is allowed to complete its action without any interference. The small dose means that it is unlikely that there will be any dangerous side effects. Hahnemann discovered that remedies can still be effective in doses or concentrations that are so small as to be undetectable. Mechanical shaking of the diluted remedies, known as 'succussion', enhances their effect although it is not understood why this should be so. This use of extremely small doses is one of the most controversial aspects of homoeopathy as it has never been proven why it works. As a result critics have labelled it no more than placebo medicine.

Homoeopathy attempts to identify the order in which symptoms and illnesses appeared, the grouping of any symptoms, and the overall relationship to the health and function of the patient. Another backer of homoeopathy, Hering, identified four symptom directions.

● Downwards from the head to the feet.

● From inside to the outside.

● From vital organs to less vital ones.

● From the most recent to the oldest, in reverse order of their   appearance.

This is known as the 'laws of cure' or 'law of direction of cure'.

Homoeopathic medicines are made into remedies by serial dilutions and shaking or succussion in a liquid or solid medium. Basic vegetable materials are crushed and dissolved in 95% grain alcohol, they are then shaken and stored. The same system is used for animal, and any other, products which are soluble in alcohol. Metals and other insoluble remedies are crushed and diluted with lactose, or milk sugar, until they are soluble. The resultant mixture is known as the mother tincture, as O, which is then further diluted with alcohol or lactose into 1:10 or X; 1:100 or C. This is then mixed and shaken and is known as 1X or 1C. The process is repeated for 2X or 2C and so on. The most common dilutions for self treatments are 6th, 12th or 30th X or C. Professional treatments use much greater dilutions such as 200C or even 1M.

Examination
Patients describe their symptoms and history without interruption. The homoepathy encourages the patient to list as many symptoms as possible and a record is made of the patients list. The homoepathy often bases the diagnosis on idiosyncratic features or symptoms which the orthodox practitioner would ignore. The

homoepathy also determines whether the patient notices any of the following:

- Any subjective sensations associated with the symptoms such as pain or anger.

- Localisation of specific symptoms such as position or side.

- Are the symptoms relieved or exacerbated by anything such as weather, time of day or diet?

- Do any symptoms appear at the same time or in sequence?

The homoepath will also physically examine the patient and carry out any necessary laboratory tests to confirm diagnosis.

As the case history is taken symptoms are assessed in terms of importance depending on how the patient describes them. The vast range of possible remedies available means that the homoepathy requires to use the repertory which is an index of symptoms and remedies which have proved effective. By identifying remedies appropriate to the main symptoms the total search is narrowed down. The remedies found in the repertory are only suggestions and the symptoms and remedies need to be assessed carefully before the final selection is made. This final selection takes into account the differences between individuals and takes into account the constitutional remedy.

Many of the dilute remedies are inactivated by sunlight and therefore require to be stored in dark, dry places. Patients are not allowed to put anything in their mouths for at least 30 minutes before and after each dose. Coffee or other foods or drinks with caffeine, such as tea, chocolate and cola drinks, can reverse the effects of the remedy and it is recommended that it is avoided throughout the period of the treatment. Other substances to be avoided are peppermint and preparations containing codeine. These substances can interact with the actions of remedies and reduce their action. The use of other herbal medicines and exposure to mothballs and other highly aromatic substances should also be avoided.

Unless absolutely necessary, as in the case of severely ill patients, other conventional drugs should also be stopped. Treatments such as chiropractic and acupuncture should not be commenced at the same time as homoeopathy. However, if they are already being used then treatment should continue.

Treatment
Remedies are available in the form of tablets of sucrose or lactose and are taken dry on the tongue or dissolved in water. They are also available in liquid form. If taken in the tablet form then they should be sucked or allowed to dissolve in the tongue rather than being swallowed. The more acute the condition is then the lower the dilution as they can be repeated as often as necessary. Higher dilutions are used by professionals for chronic or long-term conditions. Use of higher dilutions should be carefully administered and they should not be taken while their action is still in progress. The dosage prescribed by the homoepathy refers to the number and frequency of repetitions which is recommended for each individual patient. The remedy is stopped once any reaction is seen and repeat only when the reaction stops.

There are very few contraindications to homoeopathy. Even patients with severe chronic diseases or drug dependency can be offered some help. Prednisolone – which is a commonly prescribed steroid taken to relieve long-term inflammatory conditions – does diminish the effect of homoeopathic remedies. Its use, however, should not be discontinued, and this does not mean that homoeopathic remedies cannot be taken at the same time, the dosage schedule can be adjusted to compensate. Remedies are economic, safe, easy to use and have very few serious side effects. The reactions may seem unnoticeable at first, they are long-lasting and effective. However, homoeopathy is a difficult practice and even a skilled homoepathy may need to try several remedies before seeing any reaction. Since the remedies are so delicate and easily inactivated then careful precautions must be observed.

It is possible for homoeopathic remedies to over stimulate the body and produce a temporary worsening of the symptoms, which is known as an 'aggravation', a term used by Hahnemann, or a 'healing crisis'. Although this is uncommon, it can cause concern although it may mean that the correct remedy has been selected. By stopping taking the remedy, the aggravation should subside, and it can be stopped more quickly by drinking several cups of strong coffee.

Use
Homoeopathy is most appropriate for:

● Functional conditions, such as headaches, menstrual complaints or fatigue, where there is little or no tissue damage.

- Where no other conventional treatment is available. For example multiple sclerosis, AIDS, viral illnesses and traumatic injuries.

- Conditions which necessitate the long-term use of conventional drugs such as allergies, arthritis, and digestive problems.

- Conditions where elective surgery is possible but not urgent. For example uterine fibroids, gallstones and haemorrhoids.

- Conditions which for some reason have not been cured by conventional treatments.

Homoeopathy is not useful in treating long-term diseases such as liver cirrhosis or heart disease; or for those patients who require anticonvulsants, steroids and psychotropic drugs. Homoeopathy is also not an alternative to all surgery or repair of fractures.

The Future of Homoeopathy

Homoeopathic treatments are increasing throughout Europe, Latin America and Asia. Even in Britain 42% of physicians refer patients to homeopaths. As the cost of conventional allopathic medicine increases more and more developing countries are using it as a cheaper alternative.

A

Aconitum napellus

Aconite; monkshood; wolfsbane; friar's cap; blue rocket; auld wife's huid

- Fevers, illnesses and acute infections, which are accompanied by severe pain and appear suddenly or are caused by trauma, particularly in people who have previously been healthy. Often after exposure to cold and dry weather.

- Onset of colds, influenza, laryngitis, pleurisy, tonsillitis, pneumonia and other feverish respiratory infections.

- Conditions affecting the eyes, such as conjunctivitis and glaucoma, and ears, often brought on by cold and dry weather or winds. Often the affected area is sore, red in colour, and there is an associated fever. Coughs can be hoarse, dry, loud, painful and intermittent, and there may be associated anxiety as well as thirst for cold drinks.

- Other pains with sudden onset, including infective arthritis.

- Cystisis with violent pain on urinating. The urine may contain blood, and sufferers are extremely thirsty. Also urine retention after surgery, trauma or fright, as well as diseases of the kidney.

- Hepatitis with tearing pains around the liver. Again to be used when first diagnosed. Also for gallstones and diverticulitis.

● Angina with a rapid heart rate, breathlessness and a feeling of crushing pressure on the heart which gives a pain in the left shoulder, where a sudden onset is also a feature. Also right-sided heart failure.

● Conditions of the nervous system, which can arise quickly, such as epilepsy.

● Menopausal symptoms such as hot flushes.

● Some mental conditions, including panic attacks, extreme unspecified anxiety, and fear – particularly of death following trauma, during illness, or even going to the dentist – and palpitations. Also depression where the symptoms can come on suddenly.

Symptoms are exacerbated by stuffy, airless conditions, and by tobacco smoke, draughts and the cold, and are also worse at night. Things improve in fresh air and the warmth, and symptoms can also be alleviated by sitting up straight.

People who are suitable tend to be well-built and strong, high coloured and are usually healthy, but have low self-esteem and when ill may be restless, frightened and anxious. This leads to the need to prove their own worth, to the point of thoughtlessness and insensitivity. Company is sought when well, although they may have hidden fears such as large crowds of people. They believe that illnesses are all serious or fatal, and do not deal well with shocks or emotional trauma, feeling anxious and restless.

NOTES : Hardy perennial plant with dark blue flowers on tall stems produced from tubers in the roots. Found in mountainous areas of Europe and Asia as far east as the Himalayas.

PART USED: Whole plant.

BACKGROUND : Extremely poisonous. The homoeopathic remedy was extensively tested by Samuel Hahnemann.

Aesculus hippocastanum

Horse chestnut; Hippocastanum vulgare

● Constipation which features hard, dry stools and difficulty in defecation, as well as a cutting pain shooting upwards. After defecating there can be a long-lasting pain in the anus. Also haemorrhoids.

● Back pain and lumbago. Symptoms are exacerbated by walking or stooping, and pain is referred to the hips and pelvis. Sufferers may have to take several attempts to arise from the sitting position.

NOTES : Large tree which produces chestnuts. Native to northern and central Asia although now widely grown throughout Europe.

BACKGROUND : Used in herbal medicine for alleviating neuralgia, and rheumatism, as well as haemorrhoids and other rectal complaints. Also used externally to treat ulcers, and intermittent fevers.

Aethusa cynapium

Fool's parsley; dog parsley; dog poison; lesser hemlock; smaller hemlock

● Digestive complaints with violent sickness, accompanied by violent diarrhoea and abdominal pain and colic, especially milk allergies in babies and summer diarrhoea in children.

● Mental symptoms such as delirium, fits, fatigue,

inability to concentrate, and mental weakness.

Symptoms are exacerbated by heat, and are worse in the summer, in the evening, and in the early morning. Things improve when outdoors in fresh air, and when in company.

NOTES : Similar to hemlock except smaller, the plant has little, white flowers with long, thin, leaf-like bands which hang down. The plant gives off an unpleasant odour. Native to Europe.

PART USED : Green parts of flowering plant.

BACKGROUND : Poisonous, effecting the nervous and gastric systems, and causing vomiting, confusion, and fits. Used medicinally for diarrhoea and gastrointestinal conditions.

Agaricus muscarius

Common toadstool; fly agaric; bug agaric

● Disorders such as epilepsy, conditions with muscle spasms, confusion, dizziness, confusion, Parkinson's disease, DTs (alcoholism) and senile dementia. Also depression.

● Chilblains, and swollen fingers and toes accompanied by a burning hot pain and itching.

● Cramps with painful contractions, trembling and unsteadiness. The toes and feet may feel itchy as if they have been extremely cold or even frozen.

Symptoms are exacerbated by the cold, during thunderstorms, and after eating, while things improve with gentle exercise or movement.

People who benefit often are particularly sensitive to

the cold, especially when they are ill.

NOTES : Toadstool with a bright-red cap peppered with small, white flakes. Native to northern Europe, North America and Asia, where it is found in boggy areas of woods.

PART USED : Whole fresh fungus.

BACKGROUND : Extremely poisonous, so much so that a preparation of it was used as a fly killer, and is also a hallucinogen. Samuel Hahnemann tested the homoeopathic remedy.

Ailanthus glandulosa

Tree of heaven; shade tree; Chinese sumach; copal tree; tree of the gods

● Glandular fever with a sore throat and swollen, red glands which make it difficult to swallow. This may be accompanied muscle pain and a severe headache, a swollen neck, skin rash, general malaise, and headache.

Symptoms are worse during the morning, in bright light, and when lying down.

NOTES : Large tree with yellowy-green flowers (which give off an unpleasant odour). Native to China and India, although found more widely as grown in gardens.

PART USED : Fresh flowers.

BACKGROUND : The flowers can cause nausea, although used medicinally for diarrhoea, dysentery, prolapse of the rectum, and tapeworms, as well as epilepsy, asthma, and palpitations.

Allium cepa

Onion

● Conditions which produce tears and irritate the nose and throat, such as allergies, including hayfever, allergic rhinitis, and colds with bloody nasal discharge, and redness and soreness around the nose and eyes. Nasal discharge and sneezing can be worse while in a warm room, and there can be a permanent tickle in the larynx.

● Nerve pain associated with headaches, teeth and earache, particularly in children.

Symptoms are made worse by cold and damp surroundings, and are eased in dry but cool conditions. Things are worse in the evening.

NOTES : The plant grows large underground bulbs. Native to southwest Asia but now common.

PART USED : Bulb.

BACKGROUND : The onion has been grown and eaten for centuries, but has also medicinal value: a roasted onion being applied to remove the pain of earache or other conditions, and a preparation in gin used for dropsy and kidney stones.

Aloe

Socotrine aloe; Aloe ferox; common aloe

● Headache, enlarged prostate gland, prolapsed uterus, haemorrhoids and piles, constipation and symptoms caused by overindulgence in alcohol.

● Conditions with a distended and bloated abdomen, with pain in the middle of the stomach around the navel, which is made worse by putting pressure on the area. Passing wind can lead to incontinence. Also ulcerative colitis. Stools are jelly-like in consistency, and are accompanied by much mucus.

Symptoms are exacerbated by heat, particularly sunny, summer weather, and are worse in the early morning, after eating or drinking, and when constipated. Things are better in cool conditions and with cold applications, and after passing wind.

People who are suitable tend to often feel fatigued and unable to cope with the pressures of work. They can be disgruntled, angry and short-tempered, both with themselves and those around them. They often enjoy drinking beer, but it can upset their digestion.

NOTES : Succulent plant. Native to parts of Africa and probably Arabia.

PART USED : Fresh leaves are crushed and the extracted juice made into a resin which is then powdered.

BACKGROUND : Used for gastric and abdominal problems since early times, and can be used as a purgative and externally to ease skin irritation. The remedy was tried by Dr Hering in the mid 1800s as a remedy for various congestive problems.

Alumen

Aluminium oxide

● Confusional states, such as senile dementia, as well as memory loss and giddiness when the eyes are closed.

● Conditions where there is a slowness or sluggishness in the system, including constipation, poor urine flow, as well as leaden fatigued muscles and limbs. Pans and other cooking utensils made of aluminium may increase the symptoms.

Symptoms are worse when in cold conditions, in the mornings, and after eating food which is high in carbohydrates and salt.

People who are suitable are often gloomy and pessimistic, and experience feelings of impending disaster. Many have a phobia regarding knives and other sharp or pointed items, and can also have cravings for unusual things to eat, but not meat or beer which they dislike. In appearance they are often pale and thin with dry skin.

NOTES : Obtained from bauxite, an ore containing the metal.

BACKGROUND : Used in traditional medicine for indigestion remedies, where it can help neutralise stomach acid. People suffering from Alzheimer's disease have larger than normal quantities of aluminium in their brain tissue, although whether this is a cause or result of the disease is not yet known.

Ammonium carbonicum

Ammonium carbonate

● Post-viral fatigue and conditions commonly known as ME, as well as conditions where circulation is slow and the heart is weak.

● Haemorrhoids in women which bleed copiously and are worse during menstruation.

Symptoms are exacerbated by exercise, and are ·

especially bad during cloudy, overcast weather. Things improve in warm, dry surroundings, by lying down with the feet higher than the head, and by applying gentle pressure.

People who are suitable tend to be irritable and terse with people, and can be prone to bouts of weeping and memory loss. They can be heavily built, but soon tire during exercise.

NOTES : Obtained by reacting ammonium chloride with sodium carbonate.

BACKGROUND : Investigated by Samuel Hahnemann in the 1800s.

Ammonium muriaticum

Aluminium chloride

●   Conditions which feature constriction or tightness, such as colds and coughs, bronchitis, and pneumonia.

●   Backache, lumbago, and sciatica, especially when worse on the left side and in the morning, and joint and tendon conditions.

Symptoms are worse in the early morning, but also in the afternoon. Things improve after exercising in the fresh air, and in the evening and at night.

People who benefit tend to be gloomy and pessimistic, and weep easily. They can take irrational dislikes of people, and are afraid of the dark. In appearance they are often very overweight, but their limbs can be thin, and skin puffy from fluid retention with a dry scalp and dandruff. Often they have a slow metabolism with sluggish circulation, and this can result in throbbing pains.

NOTES : Compound of aluminium, obtained by chemical reaction.

BACKGROUND : At one time prized by alchemists. In medicine used to relieve colds and coughs.

Amyl nitrosum

Amyl nitrate

● Irregularities of the pulse and anxiety, such as tachycardia, palpitations, throbbing in the head, and when aware of the heart rate, especially when it misses a beat. Also severe pain and numbness in the chest, as in angina, which can spread to the arm, sometimes accompanied by hot flushes and sweats, especially during the menopause.

● Hot flushes with accompanying heat and sweat, usually because of the menopause.

Anacardium

Marking nut; cashew nut; semecarpus anacardium

● Symptoms of constriction, as if there are tight belts around the body, and conditions which feel as the digestive system is blocked and where there is indigestion, constipation, and pain.

● Rheumatism and ulcers.

● Eczema and dermatitis which is itchy and may be blistered and even ulcerated, especially on the forearms.

● Writer's cramp and cramps in the lower leg.

Symptoms are worse around midnight, by putting pressure on effected areas, and by having a hot bath.

Although symptoms can be relieved by eating, things get worse again after digestion, and symptoms are relieved by fasting.

People who are suitable often lack self-confidence and feel utterly inferior. The can be prone to mental conditions, as they find it hard to distinguish reality and fantasy, and are often forgetful.

NOTES : Tree with pink flowers, which give off a pleasant odour, and the nuts are edible. Native to Asia.

BACKGROUND : Between the inner and outer shell of the nut is a dark thick substance which irritates the skin and was used to treat warts, ulcers, corns, and bunions. Also used medicinally to alleviate disorders of the nervous system, such as paralysis, convulsions, and dementia.

Anthracinum

Anthrax

● Septic conditions of the skin, such as an abscess with burning pain. The surrounding area becomes swollen and there is a risk that the sufferer will get septicaemia.

BACKGROUND : A nosode, which is useful in treating conditions of the skin.

Antimonium crudum

Black sulphide of antimony

● Gingivitis where the gums are detached from the teeth. Also present are bleeding gums, sore teeth, cracks in the corner of the mouth, dry lips, and a salty taste in the mouth. Sufferers have a coated, white tongue.

● Loss of appetite. The sufferer feels bloated after eating, are nauseous, and are prone to vomiting.

● Corns and bunions with tender feet and pain in the heels.

● Impetigo, fungal nail infections, and nettle rash. Also warts.

Symptoms are worse in the evening, and are also bad during hot weather.

People who benefit can be quite sentimental, but also peevish. They do not like to be looked at or touched.

Antimonium tartaricum
Antimony potassium tartrate

● Conditions, such as bronchitis, where there is an accumulation of phlegm which is difficult to expel, and where breathing is laboured – especially in infants and elderly people. Sufferers may feel that they are about to suffocate, and dizziness is experienced when coughing.

● Tension headaches with a feeling like a band around the head.

● Impetigo with pustules which leave a dark mark.

● Severe back pains which leaves the sufferer in a cold sweat and makes them want to retch.

Symptoms are exacerbated by exercise, lying in a prone position, and in airless conditions, both when wet and cold or warm and stuffy. Things improve in cold dry surroundings, and when resting by sitting propped up. The sufferer may have fluid retention, the skin looking puffy, and often they do not feel thirsty.

NOTES : Obtained by reacting potassium tartrate and

antimony oxide.

BACKGROUND : In traditional medicine used to alleviate coughs and as an emetic to cause vomiting.

Antipyrine

Coal tar derivative

● Tinnitus with a buzzing sensation but with accompanying pain. Profuse sweating is also a feature, along with possible hallucinations that the sufferer is losing their sight and hearing.

Apis mellifica

Honey bee

● Conditions associated with 'stinging' hot pains, such as inflammations, redness, swelling and itching of the skin. Insect stings, nettle rash, blisters, prickly heat and swelling because of heat, and allergic conditions, including those that cause sore throats. Also inflammation of the eyelids.

● Urinary infections and renal disease with hot, stinging pains and urinary frequency, including cystitis and urethritis. Also urinary incontinence, especially in the elderly, and fluid and urinary retention causing swelling of the eyelids.

● Angina with fluid retention and shortness of breath.

● Painful inflammation of joints, rheumatoid arthritis, swollen tendons, and inflammation of the peritoneum and pleura.

● Gallstones with burning and stinging pains, as well as appendicitis.

Symptoms are exacerbated by stuffy conditions following sleep, and are worse in the early evening, and by being in hot conditions or by touching. Symptoms are alleviated in cool conditions, the open air, and by a cold bath or application.

People who are suitable tend to be hard to please, irritable, and have exacting standards. They dislike anyone or anything new, and like to maintain firm control of their lives.

NOTES : Common.

PART USED : Whole body of bee which is ground.

Aranea diadema

Papal cross spider; Aranea diadematus

● Neuralgic pains, particularly effecting the face, when onset is sudden. The neuralgia can be intermittent but extreme, with hot, searing pain and numbness.

Symptoms are worse in cold, damp conditions, and with any cold applications, but improve in warm, summer weather, and with warm applications. Symptoms are also relieved by smoking.

NOTES : Spider with a round, brown body and white spots on its back in the form of a cross. Native to many areas of the northern hemisphere.

PART USED : Whole body of spider.

BACKGROUND : Poisonous. The spider spins a web then paralyses its prey by injecting venom. The homoeopathic remedy was tested by Von Grauvogl, a doctor from Germany who was active in the 1850s.

Arbatus

Strawberry tree

● Eczema, gout and osteoarthritis: the intensity of the symptoms shifts between the skin and joints.

NOTES : Evergreen shrub with cream-white flowers and fruits like strawberries, which are edible but do not taste as good. Native to southern Europe but grown elsewhere.

BACKGROUND : The fruit is said to be a narcotic when eaten in large quantities.

Argentum metallicum

Silver

● Arthritic and rheumatic disorders, especially those of the joints of the feet and hands, including fingers and toes. Particularly useful when the pain is intermittent. Also writer's cramp.

● Other deep-seated pains in the body such as migraines and headaches.

● Symptoms of asthma, bronchitis, and laryngitis.

Symptoms are exacerbated by moving the effected joints, and are worse in the late morning. Things improve with resting the sore joints, by being in fresh clean air, at night, and by applying gentle pressure.

NOTES : A semi-precious metal.

BACKGROUND : Used in traditional medicine as an astringent and for its antiseptic properties, as well as in teeth fillings.

Argentum nitricum

Silver

● Extreme anxiety, panic, apprehension and fear associated with stage fright, going to the dentist, taking an exam or performing in public.

● Indigestion, abdominal pain, nausea, flatulence, burping and headache. Also irritable bowel syndrome.

● Urethritis with burning pains as from a splinter. Urine may contain blood, and there is also a profuse discharge. Also pain from kidney stones.

● Sore throat, hoarseness, laryngitis, asthma, conjunctivitis and eye inflammations. Also warts and period pains.

Symptoms are exacerbated by too much work, anxiety and tension, and are worse at night, and in hot surroundings. Often symptoms are experienced mainly on the left side. Things improve in cool, fresh air, digestive conditions by burping, and painful areas by touching.

People who are suitable tend to appear to be extrovert and content, are swift in movement and thought, but worry excessively about failure. Their emotions are never far from the surface. Other fears are often of dying, illness and madness, as well as of heights and crowds. Anxiety can become so strong that it causes diarrhoea. Physically they are often thin, although they prefer sugary and salty foods, but full of energy and anxiety, and may have care-worn, aged faces.

NOTES : White crystals obtained from a natural ore of silver.

BACKGROUND : Used to clean out wounds and prevent infection.

Arnica

Leopard's bane; mountain tobacco

● First aid for injuries involving bleeding, swelling, sprains, bruising such as black eyes, and pain, as well as shock of any kind. It is believed to help healing, and therefore is beneficial after surgery, trauma, and symptoms of cystitis and urine retention after injury, as well as other diseases of the kidney.

● Gout, rheumatic pain in joints, osteoarthritis, concussion, inflammations and muscle strains, as well as muscle cramps from overexertion.

● Angina where the pain involved feels as if the heart is being squeezed, and stitch-like pains which are referred to the left elbow.

● Black eyes and eye strain, as well as for skin conditions such as eczema, varicose ulcers and boils

● Halitosis, particularly fetid breath after an injury to the jaw.

● Those recovering from strokes.

● Anxiety and phobias of open spaces, being touched and approached.

● Children with whooping cough and bed-wetting following nightmares.

Symptoms are worse with heat, touch, and continued movement or exercise, although also with heat and prolonged inaction. Symptoms are eased with initial movement.

People who are suitable can be gloomy and fatalistic, and will often deny the existence of any illness, even when obviously unwell. They will avoid medical intervention, and attempt to cope with symptoms on their own. Fear of instant death, however, is common.

They do not want to be touched, and can be restless in bed.

NOTES : Perennial plant with long, green leaves, orange-yellow flowers and a dark-brown root system and rhizome. Native to central European woods and mountain pastures, although now found more widely.

PART USED : Fresh parts of flowering plant

BACKGROUND : Poisonous in large doses. Traditionally used as a poultice to treat sprains, bruises, and wounds, and low fevers and paralytic conditions.

Arsenicum album

Arsenic trioxide

● Conditions of the digestive tract, with diarrhoea and vomiting, which may be caused by food poisoning or alcohol consumption, as well as dehydration in children following gastroenteritis or fevers. Also for pancreatic and spleen disorders and appendicitis.

● Urine retention in older people, and kidney disorders.

● symptoms of anxiety, particularly when this is worse around midnight and when alone. Depression where the sufferer despairs of life but is restless and unable to settle. Also manic depression.

● Asthma, hayfever, allergic rhinitis, tuberculosis, colds and coughs (with redness around the nose, constant sneezing, and blood-stained phlegm) and breathing difficulties. These symptoms can brought on by sitting in a draught.

● Angina with a tightness of the heart and excruciating pain which goes into the back of the head, and the left hand and arm. Also left-sided heart failure, due to atherosclerosis, with shortness of breath, as well as an unusually fast heart beat.

● Stinging inflamed eyes, psoriasis, acne, inflamed skin, impetigo, boils, varicose ulcers, and dry, cracked lips.

● Morning sickness, probably with accompanying diarrhoea.

● Also shingles, sciatica, candidiasis (a fungal infection) of the mouth, and motion sickness.

Symptoms are exacerbated in cold conditions and draughts, by consuming cold drinks or food. Things are also worse in the small hours of the morning, between about 12.00 and 2.00 am. Symptoms are mainly concentrated on the right side of the body. Things improve in warm surroundings and with warm drinks, light exercise or movement, and lying down with the head raised

Those who are suitable tend to be precise and ambitious, although they are also somewhat inflexible and intolerant. They prefer their lives to be neatly ordered, are well dressed, and often thin and pale. They have an intrinsic fear of loss, including things which simply cannot be controlled, such as death, illness, financial security, the supernatural – and even the dark. Anxiety when ill is often present, as well as restlessness.

NOTES : White in colour and derived from an ore of arsenic.

BACKGROUND : Arsenic is poisonous, but was formerly used to treat syphilis.

Arsenicum iodatum

Arsenic iodide

● Allergic conditions, such as hayfever and allergic rhinitis, where there is a severe watery discharge from the nose which causes the skin around the eyes to feel burned.

● Bronchitis. The sufferer may suffer from night sweats, which they find extremely tiring.

● Psoriasis and eczema where the skin is dry and itchy.

● Hyperactivity in children.

Symptoms are worse at night, but things improve in any form of heat.

BACKGROUND : Formerly used in the treatment of tuberculosis.

Arum triphyllum

Jack-in-the-pulpit; wild turnip; Indian turnip; pepper turnip; dragon root; memory root

● Colds and hayfever, often for symptoms mostly on the left side, and where there is often cracking and bleeding of the skin around the nose and the mouth, and dryness around the lips. The sufferer feels hot and unwell, and has a copious, burning nasal discharge.

● Laryngitis and hoarseness which may be caused by overuse of the voice, as in a singer, or by exposure to the cold.

● Impetigo with pustules and blisters which may bleed and are sensitive to touch.

Symptoms are worse in the cold, especially if caught

in a bitter wind, and also when lying out flat. Things improve by drinking coffee, and are also better in the morning.

NOTES : Plant with a large, flat root and unusual leaves on long stalks Native to north America

PART USED : Fresh root.

BACKGROUND : If eaten, the root induces severe vomiting, nausea and diarrhoea, and causes a burning inflammation of the mucous membranes in the gastric tract.

Asafoetida

Ferula foetida; food of the gods; devil's dung; gum of the stinksand

- Indigestion, abdominal pain and bloating, as well as wind which has a foul smell.
- Symptoms of hysteria.
- Bone pain which is worse in the lower limb.

NOTES : Large plant with a thick fleshy root. Native to Iran and Afghanistan.

PART USED : Resin is ground down into powder.

BACKGROUND : When the root is cut it gives out a milky gum-like fluid which can solidify into a resin.

Astacus fluviatilis

Crawfish

- Allergic skin reactions caused by consumption of shell fish. Rashes are raised, itchy, and often accompanied by high temperature, chills, malaise, and swollen glands.

Symptoms are exacerbated by cold draughts, and by being in chilly conditions.

Aurum metallicum

Gold

● Heart disease and congestive circulatory disorders, including angina, where symptoms involve chest pain, breathlessness, palpitations and a pulsing headache. Valvular disease, as well as high blood pressure associated with angina and palpitations. Also rheumatic heart disease.

● Sinusitis and labyrinthitis.

● Jaundice and other liver disorders.

● Painful joints, particularly the knee and hip, and bone conditions.

● Major symptoms of depression and severe despair, even suicidal thoughts, as the sufferer feels worthless. Although they feel suicidal, sufferers also fear death.

Symptoms can be exacerbated by physical exercise, especially during the evening or at night, mental effort or concentration, and by emotional distress. They are lessened by rest and quiet, light exercise in the open air, and by bathing in cold water.

Those who are suitable tend to be excessively conscientious and hard working, and may set themselves unrealistic targets. They are extremely sensitive to criticism and prone to feelings of failure, becoming deeply depressed and suicidal.

PART USED : Fine powder.

BACKGROUND : Used from medieval times to treat heart problems, and in the 19th century to treat tuberculosis. In modern medicine used for cancer, as well as rheumatic conditions.

Avena sativa

Wild oats; groats; oatmeal

- Nervous exhaustion, stress, insomnia, lack of concentration, and anxiety, as well as other nervous complaints. Particularly useful for those recovering from alcohol abuse.
- Impotence.

Symptoms are exacerbated by drinking alcohol, but are relieved by a proper night's sleep.

NOTES : A cultivated grass. Common across Europe and north America.

PART USED : Fresh green parts of plant.

BACKGROUND : Oats are widely eaten, and can reduce cholesterol levels, as well as being used medicinally for nerve and uterine conditions.

B

Baptisia

Baptisia tinctoria; wild indigo; indigo weed; horsefly weed; rattlebush

- Severe infections such as influenza, particularly gastric flu, whooping cough, viral pneumonia, typhoid, and scarlet fever. Symptoms can often include malaise, exhaustion, confusion, delirium, and features can also be a discoloured tongue, foul breath, and stinking diarrhoea. The sufferer may develop symptoms very quickly, and sink into a stupor or want to go straight to bed. Also for salmonella.

- Gallstones with pain in the right upper abdomen which are exacerbated by walking and drinking beer.

Symptoms are worse during hot, humid and airless conditions, but improve with gentle exercise in the fresh, open air – once the person has begun to recover from the acute condition.

NOTES : Herbaceous, perennial plant with a dark woody root, small leaves and yellow flowers. Native to North America.

PART USED : Root.

BACKGROUND : Poisonous if consumed in large quantities. Used medicinally for its antiseptic value, and as a stimulant and purgative.

Barosma crenata

Buchu; diosma betulina

● Urethritis, where there is a discharge of mucus and pus from urethra. Also present may be gravel, and males may have prostate problems.

NOTES : Plant with pale-green leaves, small, whitish flowers and brown fruits. Native to parts of South Africa.

PART USED : Leaves.

BACKGROUND : Used medicinally as an antiseptic, and in herbal medicine for conditions including gravel, inflammation, cystitis, nephritis, and urethritis.

Baryta carbonicum

Barium carbonate

● Children and elderly people with conditions resulting in intellectual and physical impairment, such as Down's syndrome. In children features can include impairment of growth, and respiratory infections such as tonsillitis or tuberculosis, while in old age the condition may have resulted from a stroke.

● High blood pressure, angina, and palpitations in people old before their time.

● Impotence where the sufferer is generally sexually inactive.

Symptoms are exacerbated by the cold, in any form, especially during damp, chilly weather with a bitter wind. Symptoms are alleviated with warmth, including warm clothing, and by exercising in the open air.

People suitable for the remedy are often children, or can appear childlike, and need guided into making decisions. They can be shy, retiring and unsure of themselves, and require a considerable amount of reassurance. Feet are cold, and sweat has an unpleasant odour. They tend to catch colds all the time and feel fatigued.

BACKGROUND : Formerly used to treat tuberculosis and swollen glands, and barium is used in radiology.

Baryta muriaticum
Barium chloride
● High blood pressure, with a high systolic pressure but low diastolic pressure. The sufferer tosses about periodically as if having convulsions.

Belladonna
Belladona; deadly nightshade; devil's herb; devil's cherries; black cherries; great morel; dwayberry
● Acute conditions which occur suddenly and may involve a high fever. Symptoms include wide, staring eyes, throbbing headache, thumping heart, and red, flushed skin and face. The hands and feet may be cold, and the skin around the mouth and lips pale, but the tongue is bright, even fiery or 'strawberry' red. The sufferer may be quite hot, but does not sweat much.
● Infectious diseases such as scarlet fever, influenza, tonsillitis and sore throats, coughs, bronchitis, pleurisy, labyrinthitis, chicken pox, measles, mumps, skin infections, swollen glands, whooping cough, and at the onset of pneumonia. Coughs are dry and sound as if they scrape at the throat, and pains are tearing and

throbbing.

● Neuralgia, earache, and sinusitis with a tearing pain, conjunctivitis and glaucoma, migraines and headaches, throbbing toothache, or wisdom tooth eruption, boils and inflammations of the kidneys. Particularly when brought on by draughts or where discharge is bloody.

● Cystisis with blood in the urine and urinary frequency. Also urinary retention and pain from kidney stones, as well as kidney disease.

● Hepatitis with pain in the upper abdomen or around the middle of the stomach. Sufferers have want lemons or lemonade which eases the symptoms. Also appendicitis, diverticulitis and gastroenteritis, usually with colic.

● Skin abscess which is hot and angry, and about to burst, as well as acne with pustules.

● Infective arthritis with joints which are hot, red and tender, and extremely painful. Also inflamed tendons.

● Phobia of dogs and manic depression, where the sufferer lives in a world of their own. They may have visual and auditory hallucinations, which may be terrifying.

● Heavy periods with bright-red blood.

● Labour pains, tender breasts while breast feeding, fever and teething in children.

Symptoms are exacerbated while lying down, more intense on the right side, and are worse at night. They improve while upright, either standing or sitting, and in warm conditions.

People who are suitable are usually fit, energetic and eager, while in good health, and sociable and popular. If ill, however, they may become restless, irritable, and even violent. They may have an aversion to fluids, and whenever they swallow a spasm develops and the liquid or food is expelled through the mouth and nose. They have a tendency to grind their teeth.

NOTES : Perennial plant with oval leaves, pale purple bell-shaped flowers, and shiny black berries. Native to central and southern Europe, parts of Asia and north Africa, but grown more widely.

PART USED : Pulped leaves and flowers.

BACKGROUND : Extremely poisonous. The name means 'beautiful woman'. In traditional medicine used for neuralgia, rheumatism and sciatica, as well as conditions of the eye. In homoeopathy Samuel Hahnemann used it to treatment scarlet fever.

Bellis perennis

Daisy; bruisewort; bairnwort; garden or common daisy

● Bruising, sprains, pain and inflammation following accidents, trauma, and surgery.

● Prevention of infection and the treatment of boils and abscesses. Symptoms are worse when the sufferer becomes cold after being too hot, and glands may be swollen. Arms and legs may feel cold or numb.

● During pregnancy to relieve cramps and pains.

Symptoms are worse if cold or wet, and exacerbated by sweating, and by being too hot in bed. Things improve with rubbing or massage of the painful area, and with gentle exercise or movement.

NOTES : A common plant or weed, found in most lawns, with white flowers and yellow centres.

PART USED : Whole, fresh flowering plant.

BACKGROUND : Used from medieval times to relieve bruising, hence bruisewort.

Benzoicum acidum

Benzoic acid

● Arthritic conditions and gout, especially where there is a characteristic clicking in the joints with a severe, searing pain.

● Urinary complaints, particularly kidney stones. Urine is thick in viscosity, and smells extremely unpleasant.

NOTES : Naturally found resinous substance which occurs in some plants.

Berberis vulgaris

Berberis; barberry; pipperidge bush

● Kidney conditions accompanied by severe pain, including renal colic and kidney stones, especially where there is the production of dark-coloured urine which smells foul.

● Also gallstones, jaundice and biliary colic accompanied by the passing of pale faeces.

● Back problems with stitch-like pains in the neck.

● Warts with a burning pain which are also itchy, but are worse when scratched.

Symptoms are exacerbated by long periods of standing, and by putting pressure in the area, but may show rapid changes in severity. Thing improve with gentle exercise or movement which stretches the body.

People who are suitable tend to look pale and unhealthy, with sunken, shadowed eyes.

NOTES : Bushy shrub with pale green leaves, yellow flowers, and red berries. Native to Europe, North Africa and parts of Asia.

PART USED : Fresh root.

BACKGROUND : Used since early times to treat feverish conditions, gastroenteritis, haemorrhage, jaundice, and dysentery. In herbal medicine used as a remedy for jaundice and other liver complaints, gallstones, and digestive disorders, such as relieving constipation and diarrhoea.

Borax

Sodium borate

● Digestive disorders including diarrhoea, pain, nausea and vomiting, often accompanied by sweating, fever and giddiness. Also oral thrush with white growths in the mouth, which bleed when touched and when the sufferer eats.

● Barotrauma, a painful condition of the ears caused by a change in pressure such as experienced in a pressurised aeroplane, as well as labyrinthitis. One feature is that the condition is exacerbated by downward motion, and there is also giddiness with nausea and vomiting.

● Gingivitis with painful gumboils and a bitter taste in the mouth.

● Chilblains and skin infections with swelling of the face. Also psoriasis.

Symptoms are made worse by downward movement, such as sitting or lying down. Smoke also makes things worse, and ears are very sensitive to sound.

Bothrops lanceolatus

Yellow pit viper; lachesis lanceolatus; fer-de-lance

- Haemorrhage and thrombosis, and other conditions of the blood.
- Strokes which mostly affect the right side of the body, causing paralysis, speech difficulties, and weakness.

Symptoms tend to predominate on the right side.

People who are suitable often feel exhausted and have fatigued, weary movements. Tremor can also be a feature.

NOTES : The snake, which is greyish-brown and has a diamond pattern, is extremely poisonous. Native of Martinique, a Caribbean island.

PART USED : Venom.

BACKGROUND : Venom causes swelling and eventually gangrene.

Bovista

Lycoperdon bovista; warted puffball; lycoperdon giganteum

- Speech disorders such as stammering.
- kin problems including eczema, blisters, warts, bunions, corns, and nettle rash, especially where these weep and crust over to produce severe itchiness.

Symptoms are exacerbated by heat, and relieved by cold applications.

NOTES : A fungus in the shape of a yellow-white ball. When it is about to spore the puffball changes to brown and then ruptures, the spores being released. Native to Europe.

BACKGROUND : Used medicinally to staunch bleeding wounds.

Bromium

Bromine

● Tuberculosis, where there are enlarged, hard neck glands, especially in children.

People who are suitable tend to feel better at sea, and in appearance they are often blue eyed and blonde haired.

Bryonia

Wild hops; English mandrake; wild vine; wild nep; lady's seal; tetterbury; tamus

● Inflammation in arthritic and rheumatic disorders, especially where there is a tearing sensation, as well as sciatica, osteoarthritis, repetitive strain injuries, back problems, inflammation of the tendons, and muscle pain. Symptoms are exacerbated by movement and weather change, and in exposure to a dry, cold wind.

● Pleurisy, bronchitis, colds, influenza, chest inflammation, and pneumonia with a dry hacking cough and severe pain. These can be brought on by cold and dry weather, and nasal discharge can be increased when entering a warm room. Coughs may be dry, painful and spasmodic, and there is little sputum, although what there is quite thick. The tongue may be white, and there is a great thirst for cold drinks.

● Vomiting, nausea, constipation with hard, dry and dark stools, diarrhoea, as well as indigestion and colic. Also gallstones and appendicitis.

● Breast inflammation during breast-feeding, colic in babies, and gout and lumbago.

● Labyrinthitis where the sufferer feels better lying down but they become giddy and often nauseous when they stand up. Also travel sickness.

● Migraine and splitting headache.

Symptoms are exacerbated by movement, noise, exercise and bending, dry heat, and by lying down in bed. Things improve with rest, and gentle pressure on the sore area, such as by putting pressure on the breast bone. Things are often worse at night, after eating or drinking, and when a warm room is entered. There is often thirst for long, cold drinks. Symptoms are better when still, being left alone, and when firm pressure is applied.

People who are suitable tend to be conscientious, hard working, and dependable, but fear poverty and so measure success in a materialistic way. They do not cope well when their financial security or lifestyle is threatened, becoming worried, irritable and anxious, and even depressed.

NOTES : Perennial, climbing plant with heart-shaped leaves, greenish-white flowers, and black berries. The plant has a large fleshy root. Found in many parts of Europe.

PART USED : Fresh, pulped roots.

BACKGROUND : Poisonous. Used medicinally as a
purgative, as well as for coughs, influenza, bronchitis,
and pneumonia.

Bufo

Common toad; bufo rana

● Epilepsy, especially when the onset is triggered by
bright lights or music. After the fit, the sufferer has a
severe headache.

Symptoms are worse at night, after sleeping, and
during menstruation, while things improve in the
morning, and after resting in a prostrate position.

People who are suitable can be quick tempered,
particularly if misunderstood. In appearance they can be
quite puffy because of fluid retention.

NOTES : The toad has a mottled, warty skin. When
threatened it discharges a noxious poison, which irritates
the skin, and makes the creature inedible.

PART USED : Poison.

BACKGROUND : Poisonous, causing irritation of the
mucous membranes of the mouth, gastrointestinal tract,
and the eyes, and can produce severe symptoms. Used in
Chinese medicine. It was tested by Dr James Tyler Kent,
an American homoeopath.

C

Cactus grandiflorus

Night-blooming cereus; cactus grand; selinecereus grandiflorus; sweet-scented cactus; vanilla cactus; large-flowered cactus

- Angina, with severe pain, which is worse after exercise, and a constricted chest with a feeling of tight bands. Violent but sometimes irregular palpitations, along with dizziness, and possibly tingling or numbness in the left arm. The sufferer often experiences extreme anxiety that they are about to die, and will probably need reassurance.

- Heart attacks, with crushing chest pain, which extends to the left arm. The sufferer is in a cold sweat. Low blood pressure with a weak pulse, where there is exhaustion from any effort.

- Left-sided heart failure with rapid heart beat, violent palpitations, and particular difficulty in breathing. Palpitations are worse when lying down, and at the approach of menstruation.

Symptoms are worse if the sufferer lies on the left side, and are worse from late morning until late evening. Things are improved by resting on the right side with the head raised.

People who are suitable tend to be gloomy, unhappy and grumpy.

NOTES : Cactus with thick fleshy stems and large white flowers which exude a pleasant odour like vanilla, although they only open at night. Found in desert areas of the Americas.

PART USED : Fresh flowers and young stems.

BACKGROUND : Investigated as a homoeopathic remedy by Dr Rubins in 1862 as he had discovered the cactus produced feeling of chest pain and constriction.

Calcarea carbonica

Calcium carbonate

● Disorders of the bones and teeth, such as dental decay and caries. These include fractures which take a long time to mend, and the slow growth of bones and teeth, as well as teething in children. Also osteoarthritis.

● Headaches, eye inflammations, and cataracts which are worse on the right side.

● Ear infections which produce a strong-smelling, yellowish discharge.

● Tuberculosis, colds and coughs, often in the final stage, where crusty catarrh and yellowish phlegm are features, which is difficult to cough up at night. Symptoms are often brought on by cold and wet weather. The sufferer may feel very cold but experience a sweaty scalp.

● Hormonal conditions, such as menstrual syndrome, heavy periods with swollen breasts, and menopausal disorders.

● Eczema, skin conditions, nettle rash, nappy rash, and chilblains. Also warts and thrush infections.

● Gallstones, and kidney and bladder stones, the latter with gravel in the urine.

● Anxiety with fear of going mad or that something

bad is about to happen. Also depression where the sufferer waits around aimlessly.

Symptoms are exacerbated by damp weather, cold and draughts, and are often worse at night, when the sufferer wakes up, and during exercise and sweating – as well as being worse premenstrually. Things improve later in the morning, by bending double, and after eating breakfast.

Those who are suitable often suffer from fatigue and anxiety, and their sweat and urine can smell unpleasant. They are often short and overweight, or even obese, but are very sensitive to the cold, and tend to sweat profusely. They have an intolerance to milk and coffee, and may suffer from constipation, but enjoy eggs. Often hard working and reliable, if somewhat stubborn, they can be sensitive and get easily upset by the suffering of others. Often harboured are extreme fears of death, illness, failure, open spaces, and the supernatural.

NOTES : Derived from mother of pearl, the inner layer of oyster shells.

PART USED : Powdered.

BACKGROUND : Essential for health, and is one of the key constituents of bone and teeth.

Calcarea fluorica

Calcium flouride

● Rickets, slow growth of bones in children, weak tooth enamel, and damaged ligaments and muscles around joints.

● Lumbago, adhesions following surgery, scarring, arthritic nodules, and gout.

- Respiratory tract infections, osteosclerosis, enlarged adenoids, and cataracts with flickering of the eyes and visual distrubance which appears as if sparks are before the eyes.

Symptoms are exacerbated in cold, draughty and damp surroundings, and initially on moving or exercising. They improve with warmth, and gentle sustained exercise or movement.

Those who are suitable tend to be bright and punctual, but are a little reckless, and suffer from a lack of planning – they need advice from others to work efficiently. They may have an extreme fear of poverty and illness, and their movements are often rapid and jerky.

NOTES : Naturally occurring salt.

BACKGROUND : Found in teeth enamel, bones, connective tissue, and skin. In homoeopathy one of the Schussler tissue salts.

Calcarea iodata

Iodide of lime
- Tonsillitis, swollen adenoids and enlarged thyroid, as well as other swollen glands, and neck infections.
- Uterine fibroids, and fibrous, benign breast lumps.

Calcarea phosphorica

Calcium phosphate
- Conditions of the teeth and bones, including fractures which are slow to heal, pain in bones and teeth, teeth prone to decay, problems of bone development,

and 'growing pains'.

- Convalescence after an illness.
- Diarrhoea, indigestion, and other digestive problems.
- Tonsillitis, sore throats, and swollen glands.

Symptoms are exacerbated by a change in the weather, and in cold, damp conditions, as well as after prolonged exercise or physical activity, and because of worry or grief. Things improve in warm, dry surroundings, during the summer, and after taking a hot bath.

Those who benefit tend to be miserable and discontented with their lot, and are restless and need plenty of new challenges. They dislike routine, although they do try to be sociable. Children may be thin, sickly and pale, and are often unhappy and demanding as they fail to thrive.

NOTES : A salt obtained from a reaction of phosphoric acid and calcium phosphate.

BACKGROUND : A Schussler tissue salt, and gives hardness to teeth and bones.

Calcarea sulphurica

Calcium sulphate; plaster of Paris; gypsum

- Infective conditions of the skin with pus, such as boils, carbuncles, skin ulcers and abscesses, and infected eczema. Also present is a grey and unhealthy skin, which is cold and clammy, malaise and weakness, and yellow fur on the tongue.

Symptoms are worse in cold, wet surroundings, but

improve in fresh, dry conditions, as well as by eating, and by drinking tea.

' People who are suitable can be jealous, irritable and gloomy, and they do not like heat, even if it improves symptoms.

NOTES : Mineral deposit formed when salt water evaporates.

BACKGROUND : Plaster of Paris is used to make casts for broken limbs. A Schussler tissue salt.

Calendula officinalis

Caltha officinalis; marigold; garden marigold; marygold; golds; marg gowles; ruddes; occulus Christi; solis sponsa

● Stings, wounds, boils and chilblains, and to staunch bleeding, as well as being useful for skin tears following childbirth. Also useful to moisturise dry and flaky skin.

● Mouth ulcers, septic sore throats, and following tooth extractions, as well as varicose veins.

● Fevers, and jaundice.

Symptoms are exacerbated in damp, draughty surroundings, during cloudy weather, and after eating, but improve with walking and movement, or by keeping completely still.

NOTES : Plant with pale-green leaves and bright-orange flowers. Native of southern Europe, but now a common garden plant.

PART USED : Leaves and flowers.

BACKGROUND : Used medicinally from early times for wasp and bee stings, sore eyes, headaches, warts, and many other conditions.

Camphor

Cinnamonium camphora; laural camphor; gum camphor

● Acute conditions and fevers which feature sweating, cold, clammy, pale skin, chills, and anxiety. Also present may be very low blood pressure, convulsions, and the sufferer may collapse. Conditions include cholera.

● Used when other homoeopathic remedies have failed.

Notes : Large tree with small, white flowers and red berries. Native to China, Japan, and parts of east Asia.

Part Used : The wood is heated using steam and camphor precipitates.

Background : Used in herbal medicine for colds, coughs, fevers, inflammatory conditions and severe diarrhoea. Also used to relieve hysteria, anxiety, neuralgia, pneumonia, fevers, and heart failure due to infection. In large doses can cause palpitations, vomiting, and convulsions. Samuel Hahnemann used it as a remedy for a cholera outbreaks in the 19th century.

Candida Albicans

Fungus which causes the illness.

● Recurrent Candida Albicans or oral thrush infections.

Cannabis indica

Hashish; cannabis; Indian hemp; ganeb; ganja

● Tinnitus with throbbing, buzzing, and ringing noises, as if water is being boiled in the ear. A feature is extreme sensitivity to any sound.

NOTES : Annual plant with dark-green leaves with brownish-grey flowers. Native to India, but grown more widely.

BACKGROUND : Formerly used medicinally to reduce pain and help sleep, for some mental conditions, and for gout, rheumatism, and DTs. The plant produces an 'exhilarating intoxication'. Increasingly being accepted for easing symptoms of multiple sclerosis and other conditions.

Cantharis

Spanish fly

● Conditions in which there is stinging, burning pain, including chest conditions, such as pleurisy, as well as cystitis, urinary infections, and urinary frequency accompanied by cutting pain. There may be blood in the urine. Also for urine retention, and the pain from kidney stones, as well as kidney disease.

● Digestive complaints with burnings pains, diarrhoea, and abdominal bloating, as well as irritable bowel syndrome.

● Insect stings and bites, sunburn and prickly heat, rashes with pus-filled spots, skin infections, and scalds and burns.

● Conditions which become severe quickly, and for some emotional conditions such as irritable or violent behaviour, excessive anxiety and sexual desire.

Symptoms are exacerbated by touch and movement, and following consumption of coffee or cold water, but improve by passing wind, with light touch or massage, and are better at night.

NOTES : Derived from a bright-green beetle, which
secretes canthardin, a potentially poisonous substance.
Found mainly in Spain and France.

PART USED : The beetles are dried and ground down to a
powder.

BACKGROUND : Cure for warts, and believed by some to
be an aphrodisiac. Causes blisters if applied externally,
and if taken internally irritates the bladder, urinary tract,
and genitalia.

Capsicum annuum

Cayenne pepper; African pepper; chilli pepper; bird pepper

● Conditions with burning stinging pains, such as
heartburn, piles, diarrhoea, sore throat with a burning
pain on swallowing, bronchitis, and rheumatic disorders.
If the sufferer has an explosive cough, they can break
wind, which smells foul, at the same time.

● Cold sores, typically with ulcers on the tongue, a
burning pain on the tongue, and a rash on the chin.

● Alcohol craving which causes stomach upset. Also
present is a burning feeling on the end of the tongue.

Symptoms are exacerbated in cold and draughty
conditions, and when the sufferer first moves. Things
improve when warm or hot, and with sustained
movement or exercise.

People who are suitable are often quite unfit, as they
dislike physical exercise, but consume rich, spicy foods
and alcohol, which can make them lazy and lethargic.
They can be gloomy, and often suffer from
homesickness. In appearance they can be coloured and
red faced (although the face is cold), overweight and

even obese, and they are often blue eyed and fair haired.

NOTES : Plant with distinctive, elongated, red fruits. Native to Africa but widely grown elsewhere.

PART USED : Fruit and seeds.

BACKGROUND : Used widely in cookery, but also in herbal medicine as it produces natural warmth and aids circulation and healthy digestion.

Carbo vegetabilis
Vegetable charcoal

- Exhaustion, excessive tiredness, weakness or convalescence following an operation or illness, including postoperative shock. Also heart attacks with sudden collapse, when the body is extremely cold.
- Poor circulation, including varicose veins and ulcers, and other symptoms can include puffy legs, cold extremities, laryngitis and hoarseness, and a lack of energy.
- Indigestion, heartburn, watery diarrhoea with blood, nausea, and flatulence. Also colic in babies.
- Morning headaches accompanied by nausea, fainting or giddiness, particularly if following a large meal the previous evening.
- Gingivitis, with bleeding gums, unpleasant breath, and darkened gums. The teeth are painful when anything hot or cold is consumed.
- Anxiety about the supernatural and ghostly apparitions, as well as depression with the same fear, anxiety and irritability.

Symptoms are exacerbated by warm, damp weather,

are worse during the evening and night. Things are also worse when lying down, and by consuming fatty foods, coffee, milk, and wine. Symptoms are alleviated in cool, fresh conditions, by fanning cool air in the face, and by burping.

NOTES : Carbon charcoal derived from burning wood with insufficient air for complete combustion.

PART USED : Powder

BACKGROUND : Used for treating food or drug poisoning in traditional medicine, as well as flatulence.

Carbolicum acidum

Carbolic acid

● Halitosis which is caused by constipation.

People who are suitable often have a craving for tobacco, and also suffer from indigestion, which results in an unpleasant taste in the mouth. Their sense of smell can be very sensitive, and there is a burning sensation in the mouth that goes down to the stomach.

Carboneum sulphuratum

Carbon bisulphide

● Nerve conditions which feature weakness, numbness, tremor, and paralysis.

● Eye and vision problems.

● Wind, diarrhoea, constipation, abdominal pain, and other digestive disorders.

● Meniere's disease, with tinnitus and impaired hearing, particularly where the sufferer has or is abusing alcohol.

Sufferers may be very sensitive to the cold, have muscular wasting, and may have abused alcohol.

Carduus marianus

St Mary's thistle; milk thistle
● Gallstone colic, which is associated with a strange symptom: if feels as if a pea is being drawn through a narrow passage underneath the liver and on to the stomach. Also present is a white tongue with red edges.

NOTES : Tall plant in thistle family. Found in Europe.

BACKGROUND : Used medicinally for jaundice, gastric complaints, pleurisy, and cancer.

Caulophyllum

Blue cohosh; caulophyllum thalictroides; papoose root; squawroot; blueberry root
● Used to hasten and strengthen weak or painful contractions during childbirth.
● Absent menstruation, and conditions of the uterus, such as menstrual pain.
● Rheumatic conditions which effect the lower arm and foot, with cramp-like, stabbing, intermittent pains.

Symptoms are worse when menstruation is absent or erratic, and during pregnancy. Things improve in warm surroundings, or with warm applications.

NOTES : Perennial plant with yellow flowers and pea-sized seeds. Native to North America.

Causticum

Potassium hydrate

● Hoarseness, laryngitis and loss of voice with a dry, unproductive cough or where there is production of a small amount of thick mucus, which is difficult to bring up.

● Earwax problems where there is tinnitus with a roaring or ringing sensation which can lead to deafness.

● Cystisis with the feeling of needing to frequently urinate, but being unable to do so, followed by urine incontinence. Stress incontinence and wetting the bed, sometimes associated with coughing, sneezing, or getting excited. Also for urine retention following surgery.

● Conditions of the eyelids and face, and other symptoms can include hot pains as in heartburn, back problems, and rheumatic conditions.

● Warts which are large and bleed easily, usually found on the face and fingertips.

● Writer's cramp with paralysis of the right hand and the tongue, as well as cramps in lower limb. Also repetitive strain injuries, and rheumatoid arthritis.

● Conditions of the nervous system where a feature is paralysis on one side, or twisting and jerking movements. Also epilepsy, particularly when occurring around puberty, and stroke with paralysis.

● Depression where the sufferer cries easily and can be oversensitive about the suffering of both people and animals.

Symptoms are made worse during exposure to cold winds, by exercising, and are worse in the evening. Things improve in warm and humid conditions, by consuming a cold drink, and by having a wash.

People who benefit are often acutely sensitive to the pain of others, although they may be somewhat rigid in their views. They tend to feel the cold, and often have a weak constitution. In appearance they can be thin and pale with dark hair and eyes.

NOTES : Obtained by reacting calcium oxide with potassium bisulphate in solution.

BACKGROUND : Investigated by Samuel Hahnemann in the early 1800s.

Ceanothus

New Jersey tea; red root; Jersey tea root; New Jersey tea; wild snowball

● Abdominal pain, enlargement of the spleen, and for left-sided symptoms of the abdomen. Piercing pain is a feature which is exacerbated by lying on the left side.

Symptoms are made worse by exercise or movement, and by lying on the left side, but things improve by lying still and resting.

People who are suitable are often acutely sensitive to the cold.

NOTES : Tall shrub which has small white flowers and thick reddish roots. Native to North America.

PART USED : Fresh leaves when the shrub is in flower.

BACKGROUND : The leaves of the plant were used as a substitute for tea at one time. The root is used in herbal medicine for bronchitis, whooping cough, consumption, asthma, dysentery, and pulmonary complaints, as well as for syphilis and gonorrhoea.

Chamomilla

Camomile; anthemis nobilis

● Teething, colic and disturbed sleep with night crying in children and babies

● Menstrual problems such as heavy periods, and inflammation and pain caused by breast-feeding.

● Excruciatingly painful toothache or earache, and blocked ear.

● Digestive conditions with a sore stomach and flatulence – the sufferer feels worse after belching. Also present are restlessness and the sufferer may feel frantic. One cheek may be quite red while the other is markedly paler.

● Cystisis with a sticking pain and then burning pain on urinating. The urine is red in colour.

Symptoms are exacerbated by anger, the cold, and in the open air, and improve if the weather is wet but warm, and by fasting for a period.

People who are suitable tend to be sensitive to pain, causing them to faint or sweat, and are often women or children. They may be irritable and impatient, especially when not well or when woken suddenly from sleep. They may suffer from disturbed sleep, during which they talk or cry out while dreaming.

NOTES : A low-creeping, perennial plant with daisy-like flowers. Native to parts of northern Europe.

PART USED : Flowers and leaves.

BACKGROUND : Used in medicine since ancient times for hysterical and nervous conditions. Has a powerful soothing effect, helping to reduce inflammation, and is beneficial for eczema, disturbed sleep, and asthma.

Chelidonium majus

Celandine; wartweed; greater celandine; garden celandine

● Gallstones, jaundice, hepatitis, abdominal pain, and indigestion where symptoms include vomiting and digestive upset with a pain under the right shoulder blade. Symptoms usually occur most severely on the right side, and the effected area is sore if touched.

● Right-sided chest symptoms, pneumonia, and pleurisy with accompanying stabbing pains. One features is pain in the right shoulder blade, and sufferers find it difficult to cough up sputum.

Symptoms are worse in the late afternoon and early morning, but improve with eating, particularly hot food, and if pressure is applied firmly to the painful region. Symptoms are also alleviated by consuming hot drinks, and by passing stools.

People who suitable are often gloomy and pessimistic, and can be intellectually lazy. Hot drinks and cheese are often enjoyed, although they may have one warm foot and one cold one. In appearance can be thin and fair haired, with a sallow, yellow-tinged skin.

NOTES : Herbaceous, perennial plant with large yellow-green leaves, yellow flowers, and long, thin pods with black seeds. Native to Europe.

PART USED : Fresh flowering plant.

BACKGROUND : Used in herbal medicine to cure warts and corns, but should not be brought into direct contact with the skin. Celandine is also believed to aid jaundice, eczema, scurvy, and scrofula.

Chenopodium anthelminticum

Wormseed; Jerusalem oak

● Meniere's diseases where there is a distorted hearing pattern. Hearing is better with high-pitched sounds, while speech is quite difficult to hear. Also present is buzzing in the ears and intermittent giddiness. Another feature is a pain in the shoulder blade.

NOTES : Tree with small but multitudinous yellowish-green flowers. Native to the Americas.

PART USED : Fruit and seeds.

BACKGROUND : Used medicinally for the expulsion of worms, as well as malaria, cholera, hysteria, and other nervous disorders. The plant has some toxic effects, and causes temporary dizziness and vomiting.

Chimaphila umbrellata

Pipsissewa; pyrola umbrellata; winter green; prince's pine; king's cure; ground holly; love in winter; rheumatism weed

● Cystisis where the urine contains a lot of ropy bloody mucus, and there feels as if there is a ball between the legs. Sufferers must stand with their feet wide apart and there bodies leaning forward in order to urinate. Also prostate problems.

● Pain from kidney stones with smarting pains.

NOTES : Small, evergreen and perennial plant with dark-green leaves, light-purple flowers, and a yellow rhizome. Found in Europe, America and Asia.

BACKGROUND : Used medicinally for conditions such as cardiac and kidney disease, chronic rheumatism, scrofula, and gonorrhoea.

Chininum sulphuricum

Quinine sulphite

● Meniere's disease with violent ringing, buzzing and roaring in the ears which is associated with deafness. Standing upright is a problem, and sufferers quite often are unable to stand and fall over.

Symptoms are exacerbated by lying on the left side of the body.

Chionanthis

Fringe tree; chionanthis virginica; old man's beard; fringe tree bark

● Pancreatic disorders where there is a dull ache, occasionally a gripping pain, in the middle of the stomach. Jaundice may be present, and the liver is sore and likely enlarged. The sufferer has no appetite, and is commonly constipated. Stools are clay-coloured and soft.

NOTES : Small tree with flowers like snowdrops. Native to the United States.

PART USED : Bark.

BACKGROUND : Used medicinally for typhoid, intermittent fevers, as well as externally for wounds and inflammations.

Chloralum

Chloral hydrate

● Urticaria which is worse at night but which disappears during the day.

Symptoms are much worse when cold, and are improved when warm. Drinking alcohol makes things worse.

Cicuta virosa
Water hemlock; cowbane
Injuries and disorders of the central nervous system, such as twitching, spasms and muscular jerking, especially as in epilepsy when the head and neck are thrown back and there is a violent fit.

● Conditions following a head injury, meningitis, and eclampsia, with confusion, delirium, agitation, moaning unconsciously, and dilated pupils.

Symptoms can be exacerbated by sudden movement, and are worse in the cold, and by touching. Things improve with warmth and by passing wind.

People who are suitable often crave substances which are usually thought unsuitable as food.

NOTES : Semi-aquatic plant with large leaves and white flowers. Native to North America, Siberia and some parts of Europe.

PART USED : Fresh root.

BACKGROUND : The roots are extremely poisonous, and can cause convulsions, excessive amounts of saliva, profuse sweating, hyperventilation, and death.

Cimifuga
Black cohosh; black snake root; squawroot; rattleroot; rattleweed; bugbane; cimic; Cimifuga racemosa

- Back pain, rheumatic and joint pain, as well as sharp pain, and joint and muscle swelling.
- Menstrual and hormonal problems in women, including bloatedness, cramps and discomfort associated with pregnancy, as well as morning sickness.
- Anxiety, irritability and sadness associated with postnatal depression and the menopause.

Symptoms are worse in cold and damp conditions, when drinking alcohol, with a sudden change in the weather, or during bouts of excitement. Symptoms are eased by warmth, fresh air, and gentle exercise.

Those who are suitable are often emotionally intense females, either extrovert or introvert, who can harbour extreme fears of death and madness. These are worse during the menopause.

NOTES : Tall, herbaceous plant with white flowers on tall stems, and a dark, woody rhizome and roots. Native to North America, where it is found in woods and forests.

PART USED : Rhizome and roots.

BACKGROUND : Used medicinally as a remedy for rattlesnake poison and to provide pain relief during pregnancy and menstruation. The homoeopathic remedy was used and tested by Dr Richard Hughes, an English homoeopathist, to help headaches and back pain.

Cinchona officinalis

Peruvian bark; cinchona succiruba; chincona officinalis; china; Jesuit's bark

- Conditions such as mental and physical exhaustion

following chronic debilitating illness and loss of body fluids, including influenza or conditions akin to labyrinthitis with tinnitus. Other symptoms include sweating, chills, fever, weakness caused by dehydration, and headaches. The sufferer desires fluids during chills and shivering, rather than when feverish and hot, and they have a pallid complexion and very sensitive skin.

● Muscle spasm due to tiredness, neuralgia, nosebleeds and other bleeding, and ringing or whistling in the ears (tinnitus).

● Digestive conditions such as wind, indigestion, diarrhoea which contains undigested food, and gall bladder and spleen disorders.

● Heavy periods with dark clots of blood, pain, and a swollen abdomen.

● Apathy and loss of concentration, insomnia, and irritability which is out of character.

● Depression and associated anxiety where the sufferer has a host of worries which they cannot stop thinking about, especially at night in bed. They may feel that they would like to hurt others.

Symptoms are exacerbated by touch, in cold windy weather, especially in the autumn, and are worse in the evening and at night. Things are improved by warmth, by moving about, plenty of sleep, and if pressure is applied to any painful or tender area.

People who are suitable tend to be artistic and imaginative, but are highly strung, intense, and sometimes unrealistic. They enjoy alcohol, but dislike fatty foods and the trivial. There is a tendency to depression as they cannot follow through plans to a conclusion.

NOTES : Evergreen tree with red bark. Native to South American tropical forests, but also found in south-east Asia, India and Sri Lanka.

PART USED : Dried bark.

BACKGROUND : Contains quinine, and was used to treat malaria by Jesuit missionaries in Peru. Samuel Hahnemann tested cinchona on himself.

Cinnabaris
Mercuric sulphide
- Sore throats and tonsillitis where the throat feels constricted and closes spasmodically, often associated with those who drink excessively and smoke.

  Symptoms are exacerbated by the being undressed or uncovered.

  Those who are suitable are often fat and flabby, and highly coloured and red. Often they feel cold.

Clematis recta
Upright virgin's bower; flammula jovis
- Gonorrhoea, including blockage of the urethra and slow-flow of urine because of inflammation or scarring.
- Inflammations of the genital and urinary tract, such as urethritis and cystitis, with accompanying tingling after urinating and a burning sensation, which is worse at night.
- Eye disorders, and neuralgia.
- Dermatitis and eczema, which is worse on the hands and head, and is red, burning and scaly.

NOTES : Climbing, perennial plant, usually with bright flowers. Native to many areas of Europe.

BACKGROUND : Poisonous and when bruised can irritate the eyes and throat, and if applied to the skin produces inflammation and blisters. Used in herbal medicine for syphilis, cancer, and other ulcers.

Cocculus
Indian cockle

● Nausea, sickness, vertigo and giddiness, often accompanied by depression. Also travel sickness, especially where there is a metallic taste in the mouth, and the sufferer does not want any food or drink. Conditions include appendicitis.

● Stroke where the sufferer is paralysed on one side of the body during sleep.

Symptoms are worse during cold weather, and when the sufferer has a cold themselves. Things are also worse during menstruation, which tends to be early and painful.

People who are suitable are often quite chatty and friendly, but hate wearing tight and constrictive clothing.

PART USED : Body of the whole animal.

Codeinum
Alkaloid of opium

● Conditions where the whole body trembles and twitches, which are associated with itchiness and warmth.

Coffea cruda

Coffea; unroasted coffee

● Insomnia, especially when the sufferer cannot relax enough to fall asleep and when the brain is overactive, as well as anxiety and over-excitability. Sufferers can be highly sensitive to noise, touch, any disturbance, and even odours. Also depression where the sufferer swings from happiness to deep despair very quickly.

● High blood pressure, usually accompanied by anxiety, palpitations and trembling, where there is a sudden rise in blood pressure.

● Severe or excruciating pains such as toothache or childbirth.

Symptoms are worse in cold winds, but improve with warmth, and resting in tranquil conditions.

NOTES : Evergreen plant with shiny, dark-green leaves and white flowers. The berries, which are orange-red when ripe, produce coffee beans. Native of Africa but now widely cultivated in other tropical countries.

PART USED : Unroasted beans.

BACKGROUND : Coffee is widely drunk and can cause sleeplessness. Used medicinally for heart disease, fluid retention, and can help rheumatism, gout, gravel, and dropsy.

Colchicum

Meadow saffron; naked ladies; colchicum autumnale

● Gout and swollen joints, accompanied by severe throbbing pain. The sufferer is likely to be feverish. One feature is that the sufferer may dream of mice.

● Nausea, sickness, diarrhoea, and abdominal pains where the pain is relieved by bending forwards.
● Kidney disease with urine like ink, a condition caused by scarlet fever or similar illness.

Symptoms are exacerbated by cold, damp weather, especially in the autumn, by exercising, or by being touched. Things improve when warm and resting in peaceful surroundings.

NOTES : Plant with pale purple or white flowers and a bulbous, underground stem. Found in Europe, parts of Asia, and North America, where it grows in meadows.

PART USED : Root.

BACKGROUND : Poisonous in large doses, effecting the digestive organs and the kidneys, and can cause depression. Used from early times to help painful rheumatic and gouty joints.

Collinsonia canadensis

Stone root; horse weed; rich weed; horsebalm; heal-all

● Haemorrhoids, particularly in women, with a feeling of pain like sharp sticks in the rectum. Also present is bleeding, and alternating periods of constipation and diarrhoea with a lot of wind.

NOTES : Plant with greenish-yellow flowers and a rhizome. Native to North America.

PART USED : Root.

BACKGROUND : Used medicinally for bladder problems, gravel, and dropsy.

Colocynthis

Colocynth; citrullus colocynthis; bitter cucumber; bitter apple

● Colic, possibly accompanied by vomiting and diarrhoea, both in adults, children and babies. Also for gallstone colic and diverticulitis, as well as irritable bowel syndrome.

● Neuralgia, particularly of the face, sciatica, muscle cramps, kidney or ovarian pain with a neurologic cause, rheumatic disorders, and headache.

● Glaucoma where there were violent pains in the eyes before the development of the condition. As they eyes become hard, the eyelids begin to twitch and become painful.

Symptoms are exacerbated by anger, irritation, eating, and drinking alcohol, and are worse in cold, damp conditions. Symptoms are eased by warmth, pressure on the painful area, drinking coffee, and passing wind.

People who are suitable tend to be reserved, inflexible, and even uptight, and they can bottle-up their feelings. They are intolerant of people who have contrary views, and have rigid opinions on right and wrong. Digestive upsets and neuralgia may result from becoming angry and upset.

NOTES : Annual plant with yellow flowers and large orange-yellow fruits. Native of Turkey, but also found in arid parts of Asia and Africa.

PART USED : Ground, dried fruits from which the seeds have been removed.

BACKGROUND : Poisonous, causing irritation, bleeding,

inflammation, and cramp-like pains.

Conium

*Hemlock; spotted hemlock; poison hemlock; poison
parsley; spotted corobane; musquash root; conium
maculatum*

● Enlarged, inflamed and hardened glands, including
the prostate gland, pancreas, cancerous tumours and
nodules, painful breasts before and during periods or
because of pregnancy. One feature is beginning to sweat
just after falling asleep.

● Nerve and muscle paralysis, such as that caused by
strokes, which gradually moves up the limbs, especially
when it is accompanied by intolerance to light. This may
result in constipation with hard stools, for which this is
also a remedy. Also motor neurone disease.

● Premature ejaculation, and dizziness or giddiness,
such as that caused by labyrinthitis, which increases
when the sufferer lies down or moves their head.

Symptoms are exacerbated by suppression of sexual
needs or over indulgence in the same, or by drinking too
much alcohol, as well as watching a moving object, or by
concentrating or with mental strain. Things improve
with continual pressure applied to the painful area,
gentle sustained exercise, and with passing wind.

People who are suitable are often rigid in views and
somewhat narrow minded, with a lack of interest in the
world beyond themselves. This can cause depression,
lethargy, and boredom – sometimes as a result of too
little or too much sexual activity. They do not cope well
with long periods of celibacy.

NOTES : Tall, biannual plant with large leaves and white flowers. Found throughout Europe, the Americas and parts of Asia.

PART USED : Juice from the leaves and stems.

BACKGROUND : Extremely poisonous, causing paralysis and suppression of respiratory function which can result in death. Used medicinally to treat tumours and cancer, swelling of the joints and the skin, liver disease, and as a sedative for spasms and dysfunction of nerves and muscles. It was used to control sexual function, and – as it induces paralysis – to alleviate pain.

Convallaria majalis

Lily of the valley; May lily; Our Lady's tears; lily constancy; Jacob's ladder; ladder to heaven

● Congestive heart failure with oedema and shortness of breath, which is worse when lying down. Also increases the energy of the heart muscle, and makes pulse more regular and stronger.

NOTES : Flowering plant with long twisted leaves and groups of flowers. Native to Europe but grown more widely.

PART USED : Whole plant.

BACKGROUND : Used in herbal medicine as a cardiac tonic and diuretic, and for conditions such as valvular heart disease, cardiac weakness, and dropsy. Similar to digitalis, Lily of the Valley is weaker and does not accumulate in the body.

Copaiva

Balsam of copaiva; copaifera langsdorfii; balsam copaiba

● Urticaria associated with constipation and a fever. This remedy is particularly useful for children with a long-standing condition.

NOTES : Tree. Found in Brazil and parts of South Africa.

BACKGROUND : Used medicinally for conditions such as bronchitis, cystitis, piles, diarrhoea, and chilblains.

Cratageus

May blossom; quick; thorn; whitehorn; haw; hagthorn; halves; ladies meat; maybush

● Heart tonic, especially useful for a weak and irregular heart rate and fluid retention in the lower limbs and lungs. Also atherosclerosis and congestive heart failure.

NOTES : Woody shrub. Found in Europe, north Africa and western Asia.

PART USED : Berries.

BACKGROUND : Used in herbal medicine as a cardiac tonic and for heart problems, as well as for treating sore throats, and as a diuretic in dropsy and kidney disorders.

Crocus sativus

Crocus; saffron crocus; saffron; karcom

● Heavy periods with a copious amount of dark blood which contains long strings.

● Depression, mood swings, and weeping easily.

- Nosebleeds.

Symptoms are worse in warm, stuffy conditions, and sometimes exacerbated when listening to music, but things improve in fresh, open air, and after eating breakfast.

NOTES : Plant with grass-like leaves and large flowers. Native of western Asia, but now found in many parts of the world.

BACKGROUND : Used medicinally since early times for uterine bleeding disorders, prolonged and painful childbirth, and hysteria, as well as diseases of the liver.

Crotalus homolus
Venom of the rattlesnake

- Strokes effecting the right side of the body.
- Symptoms of jaundice and liver failure, including oedema and jaundice, as well as cancer and heart disease.
- Reduces bleeding and is used for septicaemia, shock, and collapse.
- Depression where the sufferer would like to escape from their existing lives and the people they know.

Symptoms are exacerbated by lying on the left side of the body, and by wearing tight clothing, and things are worse during warm, humid weather. Symptoms are alleviated in fresh, dry conditions.

NOTES : Poisonous snake which rattles its tail when threatened. Native to most desert areas of the Americas.

PART USED : Venom.

BACKGROUND : The venom is extremely poisonous, and

causes paralysis. The remedy was investigated in the 1830s by Dr Hering, an American doctor.

Croton tiglium
Croton oil seeds
● Copious watery diarrhoea, vomiting and colic-type abdominal pains. Stools tend to be evacuated explosively.
● Severe skin inflammations and infections which feature redness, blistering, and a feeling of heat.

Symptoms tend to be worse in the summer, and are exacerbated by touch.

NOTES : Small tree with dark-green leaves with straw-coloured flowers and fruits containing oily beans. Found in parts of India and Asia.

PART USED : Oil.

BACKGROUND : Poisonous in high doses, and causes diarrhoea and vomiting: it should never be given to pregnant women or children. If it comes in contact with the skin causes blistering and irritation. Used in herbal medicine to alleviate chronic constipation, as well as externally to relieve gout, rheumatism, neuralgia, and bronchitis.

Cuprum aceticum
Copper acetate
● Hayfever and allergic rhinitis with accompanying tears and sneezing producing a nasal discharge. Also present is a burning sensation on the skin. Coughing

produces a thick sputum which may lead the sufferer to thinking they are going to suffocate. These symptoms are associated with a spasmodic cough which can become asthmatic, and which can lead to an attack of angina in those who already have heart disease.

- Kidney disease in pregnancy when the sufferer also has diabetes mellitus. Urine smells of garlic, and also present may be colicky pains and diarrhoea.
- Cramps which are centred in the palms, soles and calf muscles.

Cuprum metallicum

Copper

- Colic-type pains in the abdomen, cramps of all muscles, and muscular spasms in the lower leg. Also diarrhoea and cholera.
- Epilepsy and nervous conditions with jerking movements.
- Respiratory conditions such as asthma, croup, and whooping cough accompanied by spasms. The sufferer main turn blue because of breathing difficulties.

Symptoms are exacerbated by hot, sunny weather, touch, and keeping feelings bottled-up, and are relieved by drinking cold fluids, by stretching, and by sweating.

People who are suitable tend to be serious and suppressed, and judge themselves harshly – and alternate between stubbornness and passivity. Young children may be 'breath-holders' who turn blue during a tantrum, while older children can be aggressive and even destructive, or prefer their own company.

NOTES : Metal.

PART USED : Ground to a fine, red powder.

BACKGROUND : Poisonous in large doses, causing convulsions, paralysis, and even death. Long-term exposure can lead to respiratory problems and coughs, colic, and wasting. Ointments containing copper were used to help healing of wounds.

Cyclamen

Sowbread

● Irregular menstrual cycle.
● Hot and searing pains in the muscles or skin, and severe migraines and similar headaches with vision disturbance.
● Cramp-like conditions of the fingers, where they have to be prised apart by force.

Symptoms are helped by taking exercise and moving around, by crying, and also improve in the fresh, open air.

People who are suitable tend to be a bit gloomy and pessimistic, and can often be depressed with deep feelings of remorse or guilt. They may desire unusual, and normally inappropriate, things to eat.

NOTES : Flowering plant which grows from one fleshy stalk with a swollen brown root. Native to parts of Europe and northern Africa.

PART USED : Sap from fresh root.

BACKGROUND : Used in medicine from ancient times to aid jaundice and hepatitis, and a regular menstrual cycle. The root is used in herbal medicine as a purgative.

D

Digitalis

Foxglove; digitalis purpurea; fairy thimbles; fairy caps; dead men's bells' witch's gloves; virgin's glove; folk's glove

● Heart disorders with as a faint, weak or irregular heartbeat which may be a feature of right-sided heart failure, as well as other heart and circulatory conditions. This may be accompanied by additional problems of the kidneys, such as fluid retention, and the liver.

Symptoms are exacerbated by eating a meal as nausea may accompany the sight of food. Things are also worse when sitting in an upright position, and by listening to music. Symptoms are alleviated by not eating, and by being out in the fresh, open air.

NOTES : Biannual plant with large leaves and a long trail of purple bell-shaped flowers. Native to Europe and grown widely.

PART USED : Liquid from fresh, green leaves.

BACKGROUND : Poisonous, but has been used medicinally to alleviate wounds and bruising, and for dropsy. Also in modern medicine for heart conditions, as it allows increased blood flow to the heart and also acts on the kidneys.

Dioscorea

Wild yam; dioscorea villosa; rheumatism root; colic root; wild yamwurzel

● Spasmodic colicky pains, including gallstone colic, bilious colic, morning sickness, abdominal wind, and diarrhoea. The sufferer often has weak digestion and a lot of wind, and pain is referred towards the right nipple.

● Other types of spasmodic pain, such as neuralgia. Also cramps.

Symptoms can be exacerbated by bending double, but improve with gentle exercise or movement, and by standing upright or by bending backwards.

NOTES : Perennial plant with long, twisted branched root and rhizome. Native to parts of North America.

PART USED : Root.

BACKGROUND : Used in herbal medicine for alleviating menstrual cramps and pain, preventing miscarriage, and also colic, particularly in pregnant women. Also useful for poor circulation, neuralgic complaints, and spasmodic asthma.

Drosera

Drosera rotundifolia; sundew; dew plant; red rot; youthwort; moor grass

● Conditions where there is a dry, persistent barking cough of a spasmodic nature, including whooping cough, with sweating, nosebleeds, nausea and vomiting, as well as tuberculosis, bronchitis, and asthma.

● Corns and warts.

● Growing pains.

Symptoms are exacerbated by shows of emotion, talking, singing, and lying down, and are worse after midnight and when too warm in bed. Things improve with fresh air, and gentle exercise such as walking, when it is peaceful, sitting up in bed, and when gentle pressure is applied to a painful area.

People who are suitable tend to be restless, stubborn and flighty, and do not like to be alone when ill. Fear of the supernatural is often present. They also believe that people are talking about them, but are withholding bad news from them.

NOTES : An insect-eating plant with leaves covered with long, red hairs. At the end of each hair is a gland which secretes enzymes which digest the insect: the leave curls over the insect when touched. Found in Europe and many other places, in marshes, river banks and other wet places with acidic soils.

PART USED : Whole plant.

BACKGROUND : Used in medieval times to treat the plague and tuberculosis, as well as corns and warts.

Duboisia

Corkwood tree; duboisia myoporoides; corkwood elm

- Eye disorders, especially for spots which move across vision in the eye, as well as painful, irritated and inflamed eyes from conditions such as conjunctivitis.
- Giddiness, vertigo, and mental confusion.

NOTES : Small tree with white flowers. Native to parts of Australia.

PART USED : Leaves.

BACKGROUND : Used in herbal medicine to aid respiratory function, to treat eye ailments, and paralysis.

Dulcamara

Bittersweet; solanum dulcamara; woody nightshade; scarlet berry; felonwort; felon berry; violet berry

● Colds and coughs, hayfever and allergic rhinitis, catarrhal complaints and conjunctivitis, particularly where the condition is exacerbated and induced by the cold and damp, draughts or sudden cooling. There is often a stiff neck and sore throat, and the back and limbs may feel painful. There is usually a profuse watery discharge from the nose and eyes.

● Cystisis.

● Eczema, itchy rashes, ringworm, nettle rash, and warts.

Symptoms are exacerbated by cold and damp weather, and during quick changes in temperature, but improve with movement and exercise, as well as warmth and heat.

NOTES : Rambling, climbing plant with purple flowers and bright-red berries. Native to many parts of Europe.

PART USED : Young shoots and twigs, leaves and flowers.

BACKGROUND : Used to treat whitlow, an abscess on the finger or toe, which was also known as felon, as well as for skin complaints, asthma, chesty catarrhal conditions, rheumatism, and absence of menstruation.

E

Elaps corallinus

Coral snake; corallinus.

● Excessive or uncontrolled bleeding, such as nosebleeds, heavy periods, piles, and strokes which effect the right side of the body.

Symptoms are exacerbated by consuming cold food and drink, during thundery weather, or by getting too hot in bed. Things are also worse if the sufferer lies on their front or walks about. Things improve during the night, and by keeping still.

People who are suitable can be excessively afraid of snakes, being alone, death, and having a stroke, as well as of the rain. They often feel chilled inside.

NOTES : Snake with bands of colour down its back. Native to Brazil and Canada, and other parts of the Americas.

PART USED : Venom.

BACKGROUND : Highly poisonous.

Epigea repens

Trailing arbutus; mountain pink; may flower; gravel plant; ground laurel

● Cystisis with a straining sensation of wanting to urinate after urination has finished. Urine is brown and contains uric acid crystals. There may be urinary incontinence.

● Kidney disease where uric acid is the problem.

NOTES : Low-growing, evergreen plant with an abundance of white flowers which have a reddish tinge. Native to North America.

BACKGROUND : Used medicinally for bladder and urinary conditions, especially when the urine contains pus or blood.

Equisetum

Equisetum; horsetail; scouring rush; pewterwort; bottlebruch; shave-grass; paddock pipes

● Irritable bladder which resembles cystitis but without infection. Other features include the bladder always feeling full and aching, and a continual need to pass urine, although only a small quantity can be produced. Also present can be kidney pain and urinary incontinence.

● Bed wetting by children, especially when caused by nightmares.

Symptoms are exacerbated if pressure is applied to the painful area, and by touching, exercise or movement. Things improve if the sufferer remains still, and lies on their back.

NOTES : Plant with long green spikes and fruiting stem which contains numerous spores. Found in Europe and in other temperate parts of the world.

PART USED : Fresh parts of plant.

BACKGROUND : Used from ancient times to help healing of wounds, and in herbal medicine for anaemia, debility, stomach ulcers, and haemorrhage, as well as dropsy, gravel, cystitis, and prostate problems.

Euonymin

Spindle tree; burning bush; wahoo; Indian arrowroot; euonymus atropurpurea; fusanum; fusoria; skewerwood; prickwood

● Digestive conditions with bloatedness, abdominal pain, and swelling of the feet and ankles because of fluid retention. Also gastritis with diarrhoea or blood in the stools.

● Confusion and irritability.

● Symptoms of angina, including constricting chest pains and breathlessness, often focused on the left side.

NOTES : Tree with clusters of dark-purple or greenish-white flowers, and bright red fruits. Native to North America.

PART USED : Bark.

BACKGROUND : In herbal medicine used as a liver stimulant, and also for scorpion or spider bites, and to help prevent gangrene.

Eupatorium perfoliatum

Boneset; thoroughwort; agueweed; feverwort

● Feverish conditions including colds and influenza with accompanying symptoms including restlessness, severe aches and pains in the bones, headache, sore eyes, hot dry skin, and little sweating but shivering. A dry painful cough may also feature. The sufferer often craves

ice-cold food and drinks.
- Pain from bone fractures.
- Bone pain which accompany conditions such as fevers, influenza, and malaria.

Symptoms are exacerbated by exercise and movement, and are worse in the morning around 8.00 am, and by being in fresh, outside air. Things improve with company, being inside, and after vomiting bile.

NOTES : Perennial plant with a thick, hairy stem and white flowers. Native to North America.

PART USED : Whole green plant and flowers.

BACKGROUND : Used in herbal medicine to aid the digestive system or, in larger doses, as a purgative. It also has fever-reducing properties.

Euphrasia

Euphrasia officinalis; eyebright
- Inflammation of the eyelids, conjunctivitis and dry eyes, bruising of or other injuries to the eyes.
- Allergic symptoms of the eyes such as hayfever.
- Cold and influenza with nasal discharge and associated with tears and redness around the eye. Coughs are often worse during the day but improve at night, although nasal symptoms are worse when lying down at night.
- Also early stage of measles, headaches, some menstrual problems, and inflammation of the prostate.

Symptoms are worse during warm and windy weather, in the evening, and when indoors, but are eased by cold applications, drinking coffee, and in half-light.

Notes : Plant with purple-veined white flowers with yellow middles. Grows throughout Europe and north America in meadows and pastures.

Part Used : Whole plant.

Background : Used from the 14th century to treat diseases of the eyes.

F

Ferrum metallicum

Iron

- Anaemia and circulatory disorders which feature tiredness, exhaustion, malaise, pallor, and cold extremities. Exercise results in breathlessness and fatigue, possibly leading to change of mood, depression, and irritability. Also anaemia in pregnancy.
- Migraines and throbbing headaches, which are particularly bad when the sufferer stoops, coughs, or goes down stairs. Also present is giddiness.
- Depression usually suffered by women towards the end of menstruation.

Symptoms may be exacerbated by even relatively quiet noises.

People who are suitable can be sensitive, restless and excitable, and suffer from mood swings, particularly when criticised. They appear to be robust and well built. They can dislike foods high in fat or cholesterol, but enjoy pickled and sour foods. An intolerance to eggs is sometimes present.

NOTES : Metal.

BACKGROUND : Important to health as haemoglobin, the pigment in blood cells which carries oxygen, contains iron. A deficiency in iron leads to anaemia, and symptoms include fatigue, breathlessness, and pallor.

Ferrum phosphoricum

Iron phosphate

- Early stages of infections, inflammations and feverish conditions, including colds and coughs, headaches, nosebleeds, bronchitis, pneumonia, laryngitis, hoarseness and loss of voice, earache, and rheumatic pains. Coughs are dry and painful, and also present is fever and a sore chest.
- Inflammation of the stomach, early symptoms of dysentery, sour indigestion, and vomiting.
- Stress incontinence which can happen with coughing.
- Anaemia during pregnancy with accompanying weakness, pallor and flushing. Also some symptoms associated with menstruation.

Symptoms are exacerbated at night and in the early morning, when hot, with violent movement, pressure and touch, resting on the right side of the body, and by using deodorants to prevent sweating. Things improve with cold applications, and with gentle movement.

People who are suitable tend to be intelligent, inventive and flexible. In appearance they can be pale but are prone to flushing. They can feel cold, particularly in the early afternoon. They may also have a rapid, weak pulse. Often present are digestive and respiratory complaints, stomach upsets, and coughs and cold.

NOTES : Obtained by the reaction of iron sulphate, sodium phosphate and sodium acetate.

BACKGROUND : Schussler tissue salt.

Ferrum picricum

Iron pictrate

● Urethritis with pain along the length of the urethra and with frequent urination at night, as well as prostate problems.

Formica rufa

Red ant

● Burning and hot, stabbing pains which may effect the joints, as in arthritic and rheumatic conditions, and gout.

● Severe headaches and numbness of the face, where the sufferer has an inability to concentrate and may be forgetful.

PART USED : Crushed body of the ant.

BACKGROUND : The ant has a painful bite.

Fragaria vesca

Wild strawberry

● Allergic reaction to strawberries with a skin rash and itching.

● Kidney stones, gallstones, teeth problems, sunburn, and chilblains.

NOTES : Low, creeping plant with white flowers and small, red berries with tiny seeds. Found in the temperate areas of the northern hemisphere.

BACKGROUND : Widely eaten, and different parts of the

plant are used in herbal medicine for rheumatic gout, diarrhoea, dysentery, kidney stones, urinary complaints, wounds, and tooth decay.

G

Gelsemium
Gelsemium sempervirens; yellow jasmine; false jasmine;
wild woodbine; Carolina jasmine

- Nervous conditions, including headaches made worse by movement and bright light, eye pain especially on the right side, and multiple sclerosis.
- Respiratory symptoms such as colds with redness around the nose, sore throat and flu-like symptoms, earache and feverish muscle pains. Other accompanying symptoms can include chills and shivering, lack of thirst, flushed face, and general malaise and heaviness. The production of catarrh is associated with warm, moist weather. Other features are sore nostrils, and possibly the vomiting of bile. The remedy is also good for post-influenza weakness, especially where features include a slightly elevated temperature, periodic chills and heats, general malaise and heaviness, and the sufferer feels as if they are wading through mud. The sufferer is also at risk from developing pneumonia, which can also be helped.
- Strokes with weakness, trembling, giddiness, and eventually paralysis.
- Anxiety associated with examinations and stage fright with trembling and shaking. The sufferer may also have a phobia about open spaces. Depression where the sufferer is broody but cannot weep even when extremely sad. Also stress incontinence.
- Some menstrual symptoms.

Symptoms can be worse in warm and humid weather, in bright sunshine, damp or fog, and are also exacerbated by smoking, excitement, stress, anticipation, fear, and bad news. Symptoms improve with light exercise in fresh air, after sweating, and after drinking alcohol or a stimulant drink. Things can also improve after urinating.

People who are suitable tend to be well built, but have a blue-tinged skin. They often feel tired and weak. Fears may control their actions, and they can be too frightened to have or enjoy a normal life.

NOTES : Climbing plant with a woody stem, large bell-shaped yellow flowers, and a rhizome with a tangle of roots. Found along the American coast from Virginia to Mexico.

PART USED : Root.

BACKGROUND : Poisonous, and can cause paralysis and death through failure of the nerves and muscles of the respiratory system. Used medicinally for conditions such as whooping cough, asthma, and neuralgic pain.

Glonoine

Nitroglycerine; glyceryl trinitrate

● Conditions of circulation and the head caused by a sudden rush of blood. Features can include hot flushes and sweats, a pounding headache, and a feeling of congestion.

● Heat exhaustion and early symptoms of heat-stroke. Conditions include angina.

● Epilepsy, as well as bursting headaches and migraines, which are likely to have been triggered by exposure to the sun. Things improve after sleeping.

Symptoms are exacerbated by heat, turning the head, and any kind of movement or exercise, such as walking up hill, and are alleviated by the cold, and by being out in cool, fresh air.

NOTES : A poisonous, clear, oily liquid, which is highly unstable and can explode. It is a constituent of dynamite.

BACKGROUND : Acts on the heart and circulation, and given to alleviate angina.

Graphites

Graphite
● Skin conditions such as eczema, psoriasis, acne, inflamed eyelids, rough dry skin conditions with blisters or pustules, and scarring. Also ear infections, fungal nail infections, thickened cracked nails, and cold sores. A feature is a honey-coloured discharge. Also bad breath, which may smell of urine.
● Duodenal or stomach ulcers.
● Cramping pains, and numbness in the feet and hands.
● Some menstrual problems.
● Lumbago where a feature is a crawling sensation over the bottom, and other back problems.
● Depression where the sufferer is particularly susceptible to music which can make them weep.

Symptoms are exacerbated by cold, draughty and damp surroundings, and with eating sea food and sweet meals. Things are also worse during menstruation, and with the use of steroids for skin complaints. Symptoms are worse on the left side of the body. Things improve with warm, fresh air, when it is dark, and with eating properly and sleeping well.

Those who are suitable tend to be unfit, and flush or sweat with slight exertion, and they like to eat well, but do not enjoy meat or sweets as this makes them nauseous. They may appear lazy and lethargic, and can be irritable, lacking the concentration for intellectual activities. Mood swings, fears, and sudden depression are often present, and they can tend to self-pity. In appearance they may be well-built although overweight, and they often have dark hair – but can have scalp conditions and flaky skin.

PART USED : Ground graphite.

BACKGROUND : Samuel Hahnemann discovered it was being used to treat cold sores and tested it as a remedy.

Guaiacum officinale

Resin of lignum vitae

● Sore throats, including tonsillitis and inflammation of the pharynx, particularly where there is foul-smelling sputum and sweating.

● Gout and rheumatic conditions with severe and stabbing joint pains, stiffness, redness, and swelling.

Symptoms are exacerbated by extremes of heat and cold, as well as damp weather, and also by exercise and movement. Things improve with rest and by staying warm.

NOTES : Large tree with blue flowers. Native of the north

coast of South America and the West Indies.

PART USED : Resin obtained from heating logs of the tree.

BACKGROUND : Used as a cure for conditions such as syphilis, tonsillitis, rheumatism, rheumatoid arthritis, and gout.

H

Hamamelis virginiana

Witch hazel; spotted alder; winterbloom; snapping hazelnut

- Piles or haemorrhoids with bleeding, varicose veins and associated swollen ankles, swollen vein walls, and ulcers, inflamed veins, heavy periods, internal bleeding, and pain associated with bruising or bleeding.
- Some headaches, and symptoms of depression, as well as impatience and irritability.

Symptoms are exacerbated by exercise and physical activity, and are worse when conditions are warm and moist. Things improve with fresh air, concentrating on a particular task, and with talking, thinking and reading.

NOTES : Shrub with grey bark, yellow flowers, and black nuts with edible seeds. Native to North America, but also grown in Europe.

PART USED : Bark of stems and twigs and outer part of fresh root.

BACKGROUND : Used medicinally to treat bruises, swelling, inflammations, piles and haemorrhages, as well as other conditions. It was tried and proved by Dr Hering in homoeopathy.

Helianthus

Sun flower; helianthus anuus; marigold of Peru

● Spleen disorders with pain radiating from the area of the spleen.

Symptoms are exacerbated by heat, but improve after vomiting.

NOTES : Very tall flowering plant with large yellow flowers. Native to Peru and Mexico but now found widely as a garden plant.

PART USED : Seeds.

BACKGROUND : Used in herbal medicine to help bronchial and pulmonary conditions, as well as cold, coughs, and whooping cough. The seeds are also edible.

Hellebore

Black hellebore; helleborus niger; Christmas rose; Christ herb; melampode

● Severe headaches where stabbing pains are a feature, which may be associated with an earlier head trauma. Also present may be confusion, mood changes, convulsions or epilepsy. Also depression where the sufferer feels black and hopeless, especially in the late afternoon and early evening.

● Kidney disease with small amounts of dark urine which looks like coffee grounds. Also present is oedema and the disease may be following scarlet fever or a similar illness.

Symptoms are worsened by moving the head, or by being in a cold draught of air, but are alleviated with warmth.

NOTES : Plant with serrated, dark-green leaves, white flowers tinged with pink, and a root and rhizome black in colour. Native to central and southern Europe and parts of Asia but grown more widely.

PART USED : Root and rhizome.

BACKGROUND : Extremely poisonous, but has been used since early times for ailments in farm animals. Used in herbal medicine for hysteria, and other nervous disorders, as well as dropsy.

Hepar sulphuris

Calcium sulphide

● Conditions where a discharge of unpleasant-smelling yellowish pus or discharge is a feature, often when the skin is sensitive to touch, including problems such as boils and acne, nettle rash, skin abscesses, tonsillitis (particularly in its later stages), sinusitis, earache, sore throat, colds with blood-stained phlegm, hoarseness and laryngitis, infected nails, mouth ulcers, pain following tooth extraction, and cold sores. Also infective arthritis.

● Wheezing or a chesty cough which may develop into a cold or flu, and for people who produce bodily secretions with an unpleasant, sour odour. This can have been brought on by cold and dry weather or by draughts. Also pleurisy.

Symptoms seem worse when conditions are cold and dry, particularly when undressing during the winter, when caught in draughts, and when touched. Things improve when warm, by covering the head, and after eating a meal.

People who are suitable tend to be difficult to please, easily offended and irritable, particularly when ill. They are often overweight and lethargic, with pale skin, and can be disconsolate and depressed, acutely feeling the symptoms of their condition. Outer calmness may mask anxiety and restlessness. They may feel that life has treated them harshly.

BACKGROUND : Applied externally to treat swellings caused by tuberculosis, gout, rheumatism and goitre, as well as itching skin. It was tried and proved by Samuel Hahnemann as a remedy for the poisonous effects of mercury – which was then widely used by physicians.

Hydrastis canadensis
Golden seal; yellow puccoon; Indian dye; orange root; eye balm; eye root; ground raspberry
● Infections of the chest, throat and nose which feature the production of a thick, yellow catarrh, along with a sore throat and other pains.
● Digestive disorders which feature constipation, nausea, vomiting, and loss of appetite and weight. Useful for people who have lost a lot of weight because of a long illness, as well as for hepatitis.

Symptoms are worse during the evening and at night, and out in cold air, but things improve with heat, and in tranquil, warm surroundings.

NOTES : Small, perennial plant with green-white flowers, an inedible fruit which resembles a raspberry, and a rhizome and tangled root system. Native to parts of North America.

PART USED : Rhizome.

BACKGROUND : Used medicinally for digestive complaints, liver conditions, eye irritations, ulcers and cancers, and conditions where catarrh is a feature. The homoeopathic remedy was tested by Dr Hale in 1875.

Hyoscyamus

Henbane; hyoscyamus niger; henbell; hogbean

●   Paranoia, jealousy and unreasonable behaviour, aggressive outbursts and use of foul language with sexual swear words. Also manic depression where the sufferer may be very suspicious and jealous of others.

●   Muscular spasms and crampy, intermittent pains, which may accompany epilepsy, as well as disorders of the digestive system and bladder. Also Parkinson's disease.

●   Alcoholism with accompanying hiccups and sometimes vomiting which may contain blood.

Symptoms are exacerbated by lying down, and when suffering from emotional upsets, but are alleviated by sitting in an upright position.

People who are suitable can be talkative and make jokes, laughing at anything, but are also suspicious.

NOTES : Both annual and biannual plant. Found in many parts of the world.

PART USED : Juice from whole, fresh, flowering plant.

BACKGROUND : Extremely poisonous, but used from early times to alleviate pain and induce sleep. Used in herbal medicine for nervous conditions, asthma, irritable cough, irritable bladder, and stomach ulcers. Also given to aid insomnia.

Hypericum

St John's Wort

● Conditions with stabbing or shooting pains associated with trauma and nerve damage, including conditions of the spinal cord, head or eye injuries, and concussion.

● Wounds, crushing injuries and lacerations, and for bites, stings, puncture wounds, splinters, and pain following tooth extraction.

● Nausea, sickness and indigestion, as well as asthma, haemorrhoids or piles, and some menstrual problems, with an accompanying headache.

Symptoms are exacerbated by cold or damp weather, and are worse before a thunder storm, and after getting cold while preparing for bed. Things are also worse in close, stuffy conditions and when touched. Symptoms are eased by not moving, and when the head is tilted backwards.

NOTES : Perennial, herbaceous plant with dark-green leaves, which have oil-secreting glands, and bright-yellow flowers. Native of Europe and Asia, where it is found in woods, meadows and hedges.

PART USED : Whole plant including flowers.

BACKGROUND : The ground flowers produce a blood-red juice, which was used to treat wounds, and the plant was believed to protect against evil. It has many medicinal uses, such as bladder complaints, diarrhoea, jaundice, nervous depression, and haemorrhages.

I

Iberis amara
Bitter candytuft
● Angina, palpitations which can be violent and are induced by the slightest effort, breathlessness, chest pains, and oedema. Other heart conditions, including left-sided heart failure. A feature is that the sufferer wakes up around 2.00 am with palpitations. The windpipe is filled with mucous, resulting in breathing difficulties and coughing that makes the sufferer go red in the face.
● Bronchitis, asthma, sickness, and vertigo.

Symptoms are exacerbated by lying down, especially by lying on the left side.

NOTES : Small, annual plant with milky-white flowers. Found in much of Europe.

PART USED : Seeds.

BACKGROUND : Used in herbal medicine for gout, rheumatism and associated conditions, dropsy, asthma and bronchitis. The homoeopathic remedy was tested by Dr Edwin Hale, an American homoeopath.

Ignatia
Ignatius bean; strychnos ignatii; ignatia amara
● Symptoms of shock, bereavement, grief and loss, especially when the sufferer is finding it hard to come to

terms with a traumatic event. Accompanying symptoms can include hysteria, cramps, anger, and lack of sleep. Also night crying in babies, who may have picked up their mother's own grief reaction.

● Anxiety, phobias and fear, especially when accompanied by depression, self-doubt, pity, blame, and fits of weeping. Depression with mood swings but where the sufferer can be quite broody and uncommunicative.

● Tension headaches and digestive problems such as diarrhoea with colic, feverish symptoms and chills, and pain in the abdomen. Also colic in babies.

● Tonsillitis and sore throat, especially when the tonsils are ulcerated.

● Some problems associated with menstruation, such as sharp pains or absence of periods.

● Enlargement of the spleen. Symptoms are lessened by lying on the left side, even although this is the side of discomfort.

● Epilepsy where the condition is brought by great grief or fear.

Symptoms are worse in cold weather and surroundings, by being touched, and are exacerbated by smoking, or drinking coffee. Things improve with warm conditions, light exercise and moving about, eating, after passing urine, and with lying on the side or area which is painful.

Those who are suitable tend to be women who are self critical and sensitive, but also artistic and intelligent. They may hide their emotions and worry excessively about rejection, and can be claustrophobic and sensitive to pain. Mood swings are a common feature. They often find that alcohol, sweets and fruit upset the digestion, while sour foods, bread and dairy products are enjoyed. They are prone to sighing, yawning, and excessive blinking. In appearance they may be dark haired and slim, but often have a worried expression.

NOTES : Woody, climbing shrub with white flowers which produce seed pods. Native to the Philippines and parts of Asia.

PART USED : Powdered seeds.

BACKGROUND : Pods contain strychnine, which disrupts the nervous system, and are extremely poisonous. The tree is called after Ignatius Loyola, who was the founder of the Jesuit Order in the early 16th century, as the Jesuits brought seeds of the tree back to Europe. The beans were used as a remedy for cholera, and for some heart complaints.

Iodum

Iodine

● Hyperthyroidism, features of which include weakness and wasting, particularly in the limbs, excessive hunger, cutting pains, pain and bulging of the eyes, restlessness, nervousness and sweating, breathlessness, rapid heart beat, and intolerance to heat.

● Other conditions with the same symptoms, such as pancreatic disorders.

● Disorders of the spleen with pain and tenderness.

● Severe hacking coughs, laryngitis and other throat problems, breathlessness, tuberculosis, and pain in the bones.

● Anxiety associated with the self and current

situations. Also depression where the sufferer may act irrationally and do something violent, such as killing themselves or others.

Symptoms are exacerbated by heat, and are alleviated by cool, fresh air, as well as by exercising and moving, and after eating meals.

People who benefit are often busy, and they tend to be excitable and very talkative. Although they eat well, a quick metabolism means that they can quickly lose weight. They can, however, be quite forgetful, inefficient and disorganised, and get quite easily fatigued. In appearance they often have dark hair and complexion.

NOTES : Brown, liquid element which is found in table salt.

BACKGROUND : Necessary for normal functioning of the body, and is a major part of thyroid hormones, which regulate many body processes. Iodine deficiency can cause mental and physical fatigue, weight gain, swelling of the face and neck, and a dry skin.

Ipecacuanha

Cephaelis ipecacuanha; Psychotria ipecacuanha; ipecac root
● Conditions where the main symptoms are persistent nausea and vomiting, such as morning sickness and motion sickness, as well as conditions such include inflamed salivary glands. Also present may be diarrhoea which smells foul and has a lot of undigested food.
● Respiratory illnesses such as colds, asthma,

bronchitis, whooping cough, and breathlessness caused by fluid in the lungs, as well as heart failure, especially when associated with vomiting. Often it is difficult to produce much mucus even when coughing. This remedy is particularly useful for children and babies.

● Epilepsy which mainly effects the left side and where there is accompanying nausea and possibly vomiting.

● Heavy periods with a copious amount of bright-red blood and nausea.

Symptoms are exacerbated by cold weather, lying down, and after a meal which consists of pork or veal. Things improve with fresh air, and while resting with eyes closed.

NOTES : Plant with a thin stem. Native to parts of South America.

PART USED : Root.

BACKGROUND : Used medicinally as a cure for dysentery, as well as for aiding digestion, colds and coughs.

Iris versicolor

Blue flag; iridacae; water flag; poison flag; liver lily; flag lily; snake lily; dagger flower; dragon flower

● Indigestion, vomiting, nausea, diarrhoea, and colicky pains, often involving cutting pains and a burning in the stomach. This includes disorders of the pancreas, and enlargement of the thyroid gland.

● Migraine headaches where the pain is on the right-hand side, the onset of which is caused by resting after a period of intense concentration.

● Swollen salivary glands with a copious production of saliva.

Notes : Plant with deep-blue flowers and a rhizome. Native to North America but now grown widely in gardens.

Part Used : Rhizome.

Background : Extremely poisonous, causing sickness and diarrhoea. Used in herbal medicine to predict disorders of the liver and duodenum, as well as a blood purifier. Also to treat scrofula, syphilis, dropsy, and skin conditions.

J

Juniperus communis
Juniper; genevrier; ginepro; enebro

● Kidney disease, especially in the older sufferer who has had repeated attacks. Urine smells of violets.

NOTES : Shrub with flowers and berries. Found in many parts of the northern hemisphere.

PART USED : Berries.

BACKGROUND : Used in herbal medicine to help indigestion, wind, and dropsy as well as kidney and bladder conditions. The berries are used to flavour gin.

K

Kali arsenicum

Fowler's solution

- Eczema where the skin in the bends of the elbow and knees has a tendency to develop cracks. Also psoriasis with extreme itchiness.
- Anxiety with where the sufferer is easily startled.

Symptoms are exacerbated by undressing, and are worse in warm surroundings, and when walking.

People who benefit are often quite nervous, and can be anaemic.

Kali bichromicum

Potassium bichromate

- Conditions which involve mucus membranes, particularly where there is an unpleasant-smelling discharge, including the vagina, genital and urinary tracts, throat, nose, and stomach and gall bladder.
- Colds and sinusitis, particularly where there are crusts of catarrh and a yellowish-greenish, foul-smelling discharge which is ropy in nature – the nose may be red and sore. Headache, migraine, and glue ear as well as feelings of fullness and pressure.
- Joint, back and rheumatic conditions with pain that may be experienced in different areas and even stop suddenly. Sciatica which is worse when the sufferer urinates. Also varicose ulcers.

Symptoms are exacerbated in hot, sunny surroundings, particularly during the summer, and when ill, cold or chilled, or after drinking alcohol, particularly beer. Things are also worse in the small hours of the morning, and on first awakening. Symptoms are eased by moving around and with light exercise, after eating, and after vomiting. Things also improve with warmth and heat, although not hot sun, as well as by undressing.

People who are suitable tend to be inflexible and rigid: those whose lives are bound by routine. They can be fussy and imprecise, conformist, and very law-abiding.

NOTES : Bright, orange crystals.

Kali bromatum

Potassium bromide

● Skin disorders such as severe acne and psoriasis, especially where the sufferer is feeling weak, both mentally and physically.

● Excessive menstrual bleeding, especially during the menopause.

● Depression where the sufferer may become paranoid, believing that they are to be poisoned or are being followed. Also manic depression where the sufferer may feel they are being punished by God, and they suffer from night terrors.

Symptoms are worse during menstruation, and thing improve when fully occupied.

People who are suitable need to keep occupied, and tend to be restless and anxious. During their adolescence they can feel guilty and nervous about their emerging sexuality, and they require a lot of care and reassurance. Many have strong religious feelings which makes them believe that their sexual desires are immoral, which leads to stress and internal conflict. They can be prone to acne, especially at puberty and during times of hormonal change.

NOTES : White, crystalline substance.

BACKGROUND : In traditional medicine used to reduce sexual drive, as well as for some psychiatric disorders and epilepsy

Kali carbonicum

Potassium carbonate

● Conditions of mucous membranes of the upper respiratory tract and digestive organs. Coughs and bronchitis with stitch-like or cutting pains, and sometimes lumps of blood-stained mucus, tonsillitis and sore throats, menopausal and menstrual problems, and pains in the back and the head. Fluid retention is also a feature, which causes swelling in the face and especially in the eyelids. The symptoms make the sufferer particularly prone to catching colds or flu, and they often feel chilled.

● Gallbladder conditions, possibly with jaundice. Also present many be wind, and a craving for sugary foods, and symptoms are exacerbated by eating fatty food.

● Warts which itch.

● Anxiety associated with being alone.

Things are worse in the early morning, around 3.00 am, and when it is cold, but are better in warm, dry conditions and weather. Asthmatic coughs can be relieved by leaning forward so the head is on the knees.

People who are suitable can be jealous and possessive, and can be difficult to live with. They tend to be inflexible with a strict sense of duty, and rigid ideas about what is right and wrong. They do not cope well with receiving bad news or any kind of emotional trauma, and may feel as if they have been hit in the abdomen.

BACKGROUND : Essential to good health.

Kali iodatum

Potassium iodide

● Colds with redness around the nose, sore throats, sinusitis, hayfever, flu-like infections, catarrh in chesty conditions, and swollen glands, particularly where there is a yellow-green discharge. The nose is red and sore, and eyes smart and produce tears. A frontal headache may also be a feature, as is extreme thirst. The sufferer may suffer from being hot and cold, and being drenched in sweat.

● Prostate disorders.

● Swollen painful knee joints, and inflammations of the tendons.

Things are exacerbated by touch and heat, and are worse in the early hours of the morning. Symptoms improve with moving about and when in cool, fresh air.

People who are suitable are often dogmatic, irritable and bad-tempered, and can be difficult to get along with.

NOTES : The compound is formed by reacting potassium

hydroxide with iodine.

BACKGROUND : Formerly used to treat syphilis. Potassium is sometimes added to animal feed and salt to prevent deficiency in iodine.

Kali muriaticum

Potassium chloride

● Inflammations and infections of the mucous membranes with production of a thick, mucous discharge, such as middle ear and throat infections, glue ear in children, and tonsillitis. Also present can be a very sore throat, which makes swallowing painful and difficult, fever, and swollen glands.

Symptoms are worse in cold air, either damp or fresh, and exacerbated by eating fatty foods, and during menstruation. Things are better for gently rubbing the painful area, and by sipping cold drinks.

NOTES : White or colourless crystalline substance.

BACKGROUND : Schussler tissue salt. Deficiency can effect the capacity of the blood to clot.

Kali phosphoricum

Potassium phosphate

● Conditions which feature exhaustion, weakness, and possible paralysis, such as post-viral fatigue syndrome and the condition commonly known as ME, especially in young people who have been overworked. Symptoms can include extreme muscular fatigue, being startled by a loud noise or other interruption, gloominess, depression, and desire for solitude. There may also be a discharge, containing pus, from the lungs, bowels, vagina or bladder. This can be accompanied by anxiety, insomnia, sweating after eating or when excited, tremors, and excessive hunger pains.

● Depression which may be caused by business or financial worries.

Symptoms are exacerbated by anxiety, by consuming cold drinks, and during cold dry weather, particularly in the winter. Things are also made worse by noise, strenuous exercise, animated conversation, and by touch. Symptoms are eased by gentle movement, after eating a nutritious meal, when warm, and during cloudy weather.

Those who are suitable tend to be extrovert and sure of themselves, but can become quickly exhausted. They may be very sensitive, taking bad news hard, even when it does not concern them directly. They often crave sweet foods, while not enjoying bread.

NOTES : Obtained by reacting dilute phosphoric acid with a solution of potassium carbonate.

BACKGROUND : Essential for the normal functioning of nerve tissue. A Schussler tissue salt.

Kali sulphuricum

Potassium sulphate

● Conditions with a thick white or yellow discharge, including bronchitis and infections of the nose and throat.

● Skin problems with a pus-like discharge or profuse flaking of the skin, including psoriasis and eczema, as well as measles and scarlet fever, and rheumatism.

Symptoms are exacerbated by hot conditions, and are alleviated by the cold, and by being in cool, fresh air.

BACKGROUND : Schussler tissue salt.

Kalmia latifolia

Mountain laurel; broad-leaved laurel; sheep laurel; calico bush; lambkill; kalmia

● Symptoms which predominate on the right side of the body, such as facial and other neuralgia, shingles, rheumatic pains, numbness and paralysis, and heart problems such as angina and rheumatic heart disease. Pain is sharp and shoots through the body. Heart disease may be associated with a rheumatic complaint.

Symptoms are made worse by cold, but are alleviated by warmth.

NOTES : Large, evergreen shrub with pink flowers and berries. Native to parts of the United States.

PART USED : Fresh leaves.

BACKGROUND : Poisonous, but was used by Native Americans and others to treat skin diseases, fevers, syphilis, neuralgia, blood disorders, haemorrhages, diarrhoea, and dysentery.

Kreosotum

Croesote in spirits

● Infections where pus or other discharges with a foul smell are a feature. Skin eruptions, boils, gum disease, and tooth decay with bad breath. Also rapid tooth decay of the first teeth in children, and gingivitis with bleeding, discoloured gums, bad breath, and painful teeth with black spots.

●   Infections of the uterus, bladder, pelvic organs and prostate gland. Also present can be debility and general fatigue, as well as nausea, vomiting, diarrhoea, and colicky pains.

Symptoms may predominate on the left side.

L

Lac caninum

Milk from a bitch

● Erosion of the cervix, in which the cells which line the womb are worn away.

● Sore breasts during breast feeding or before menstruation.

● Sore throats such as tonsillitis, as well as for diphtheria.

● Anxiety where the sufferer feels as if they are going to faint. Also depression where the sufferer is full of fear, and feel that they cannot contain all their feelings and need to scream.

Symptoms are exacerbated by touch or pressure, but are better when out in the open air.

People who are suitable can be highly sensitive, timid, forgetful and prone to letting imagined fears run away with them. In contrast they can also be difficult and aggressive. Nightmares are common, and many have excessive fears, including phobia of snakes. They often enjoy spicy, salty food and hot drinks.

BACKGROUND : Used from ancient times for ear infections, sensitivity to light, and female reproductive disorders.

Lachesis

Venom of the bushmaster or surukuru snake;
Trigonocephalus lachesis; Lachesis muta

- Varicose veins and ulcers, and other problems of circulation characterised by a bluish tinge to the skin.

- Weak heart or angina, as well as palpitations, cramp-like pain, and an irregular, fast or weak pulse – other symptoms may include chest pain, a suffocating cough, and difficulty in breathing. Also for dissolving blood clots, and left-sided heart failure.

- Conditions of the uterus, especially premenstrual congestion and pain that subsides when periods start. Also as menopausal problems, particularly hot flushes.

- Headaches and stroke, especially when these are focused on the left side, as well as deep vein thrombosis, nosebleeds, bleeding piles, problems of the rectum and bladder, ulcers, and slowly healing wounds.

- Vomiting because of appendicitis and digestive disorders, sore throats and throat conditions, ear wax problems, bronchitis, laryngitis caused by overuse of the voice, and lung abscess.

- Boils, acne, shingles, skin infections and ulcers, and fevers with chills and shivering.

- Jaundice with a swollen abdomen, and kidney stones.

- Nervous conditions with jerking of the sufferer's limbs. Also alcoholism.

- Severe symptoms of measles, scarlet fever and smallpox.

- Depression where the sufferer become obsessed with religious worries, and may feel that friends and family are planning their funeral.

Symptoms are exacerbated by touch, pressure, and particularly tight clothing, and are worse after sleeping, as well as in hot sun or in a hot bath, after consuming hot food or drinks. Things are also worse during the menopause. Symptoms are lessened when out in fresh air, drinking cold drinks, and for the discharging normal body excretions. Chest symptoms are alleviated by sitting up and bending forward.

Those who are suitable are intelligent, ambitious, and creative, although they can be somewhat intense, opinionated and impatient. They find it difficult to commit themselves to a relationship. The tend to enjoy pickled foods, rice, bread, oysters, coffee, and alcohol, although hot drinks and wheat-based foods do not agree with them. They are prone to fears, including of water, suffocating, strangers, being burgled, and dying. They can be prone to being overweight, and ginger haired with freckles; alternatively they are sometimes pale but dark haired, thin, but with a lot of energy, although there may be a bluish tinge to their skin. Children who benefit may be possessive of their friends, and this jealousy can lead to being naughty.

NOTES : Venom of the bushmaster snake. Native to South Africa.

BACKGROUND : Extremely poisonous. Wounds bleed copiously and there is also a risk of haemorrhaging, as well as of blood poisoning or septicaemia. Investigated as a homoeopathic remedy by Dr Constantine Hering.

Lathyrus

Chick pea

● Paralysis of the lower limbs with stiffness, pain and exhaustion, such as in poliomyelitis and multiple sclerosis.

BACKGROUND : Used for culinary purposes and the

Latrodectus mactans

Female black widow spider

● Serious heart complaints, such as heart attack and angina, with extreme chest pain which goes into the left armpit and into the left arm down to the fingertips. The arm feels as if it is paralysed. Pulse is weak and rapid.

● Anxiety states and fear, accompanied by hyperventilation, agitation, breathlessness, and collapse.

Symptoms are worse during cold, damp conditions, and in thundery weather. Things are also worse at night, but are better with reassurance, sitting still, and by taking a hot bath.

PART USED : Body of spider.

BACKGROUND : The venom causes constricting chest pains, sweating, spasm in muscles and blood vessels, fear, collapse, and death.

Laurocerasus

Cherry laurel; prunus laurocerausus; cherry bay; common laurel

● Breathlessness and cyanosis, a blue tinge to the skin because of a lack of oxygen, with a spasmodic cough.

The symptoms are as a result of a serious disorder of the lungs or heart, such as left-sided heart failure where the sufferer, who is very breathless, clutches at the heart. Symptoms are worse when sitting up.

NOTES : Small, evergreen shrub with dark, shiny leaves, white flowers, and black, cherry-like fruits. Native to parts of Asia but more widely grown in gardens.

PART USED : Fresh leaves.

BACKGROUND : Used in herbal medicine to treat whooping cough and asthma. The leaves give off a bitter almonds smell because of prussic acid .

Ledum

Marsh tea; wild rosemary; ledum palustre

- First aid remedy for insect stings, animal bites, lacerations, and wounds with bruising and stabbing or sharp pains. This is often accompanied by inflammation, swelling, and redness, and can also include feverish symptoms, such as shivering and feeling chill.
- Rheumatic pain in the feet which radiates upwards, painful and hot-feeling joints and tendons with accompanying stiffness but with cold-feeling skin, gout in the big toe, and muscular stiffness. Also osteoarthritis.
- Cataracts, particularly in those suffering from gout.

Symptoms are exacerbated when in warm or hot conditions, during the night, and when touched. Things improve with cold applications to the sore area, and in cool surroundings.

People who are suitable are prone to be sweaty at night when ill. They tend to have itchy skin on their

lower leg and feet, and can be prone to spraining their
ankles. They may be irritable and hard to please when
sick, and often want to be left by themselves.

NOTES : Evergreen shrub with long, dark-green leaves
and white flowers. Native to areas of northern Europe,
North America, and parts of Asia.

PART USED : Fresh parts of plant, then dried and
powdered.

BACKGROUND : Used by folk living in Scandinavia to
repel insects and mice. The flowers are believed to have
antiseptic properties.

Lilium tigrinum

Tiger lily

● Disorders of the female reproductive organs,
including a prolapsed uterus with dragging pains,
uterine fibroids which may effect the bladder increasing
the desire to urinate, swollen ovaries and ovarian pain,
and itching in the genital region.

● Disorders of the bladder, rectum and veins, and for
symptoms of angina, such as severe constricting pain –
the heart feeling as if is gripped in a vice, anxiety, rapid
palpitations, and rapid heart rate, and numbness
extending down the right arm.

● Depression where the sufferer is consumed with the
idea they are about to get a life-threatening illness.

Symptoms are exacerbated by heat, and are worse at
night, and in a crowded room. Things are better in cool
conditions, and when out in cold, fresh air, and are
alleviated by lying on the left side.

People who are suitable have a high moral sense and set themselves very high standards. This can result in conflict between sexual desires and behaving in what is perceived as the correct manner, and can result in self-disgust and extreme guilt. This conflict can also lead to irritability and being over-sensitive to critical remarks. They tend to have hot hands, and prefer cold or cool weather and conditions.

NOTES : Perennial, aquatic plant with large orange funnel-shaped flowers and petals have deep-red spots. Native to China and Japan but widely grown in gardens.

PART USED : Fresh flowering plant.

BACKGROUND : Used medicinally for dysentery, diarrhoea, gonohorrea, boils, tumours, and skin conditions. The homoeopathic remedy was tested by the American homoeopathist Dr Carroll Dunham in 1869.

Lithium carbonicum

Lithium carbonate

- Gallbladder conditions, where there are violent pains in the area of the liver, and also in the bladder. The sufferer tends to have a red nose.
- Kidney stones with pain in the heart area when urinating or bending over. The pain is colicky and usually focused on the right side around the kidney.

BACKGROUND : Used in traditional medicine for manic depression.

Lycopodium

Club moss; lycopodium clavatum; wolf's claw; vegetable sulphur; stag-horn's moss; running pine

● Conditions of digestion and the kidney, including indigestion, heartburn, sickness, nausea, wind, bloatedness, and constipation, as well as appendicitis.

● Cystisis where it takes a long time to urinate and the urine may contain a red sediment, as well as urinary frequency and incontinence. Also urine retention, and pain from kidney stones.

● Bleeding haemorrhoids and piles.

● Right-sided symptoms, as well as nettle rash, psoriasis affecting the hands, fatigue because of illness, and ME-type conditions, some headaches, coughs, bronchitis, rhinitis, glue ear, and sore throats. Chest symptoms feature constricting pain whenever the sufferer coughs, and sputum is thick, blood stained and has a salty taste.

● Gout and recurrent arthritis.

● Relieving distress caused by anxiety, fear, and apprehension associated with insecurity and stressful events, such as examinations or stage fright. Also for premature ejaculation and those unable to sustain an erection.

● Insomnia, talking during sleep, night terrors, and fear when first waking up. Also depression where the suffer finds it hard to cope when on their own and loses self esteem.

Symptoms predominate on the right side, and seem worse in late afternoon and early evening, between about 4.00 and 8.00 pm. Things are also worse when in warm and stuffy conditions, wearing clothes which are too constricting, during the spring, and after eating too much. Symptoms are relieved in outdoor, fresh and cool conditions, with loosening tight clothing, after consuming hot food or drink, with light exercise, and at night.

People who are suitable tend to be hard-working, intelligent, and slightly serious. They may appear to be confident but this can mask a lack of self-worth. They can be sexually promiscuous and do not like commitment. They are often unsympathetic with illness. They enjoy sweet foods and hot meals and drinks, and although they can become full quickly, they may continue eating and drinking. Fear of being alone, failure, darkness, crowds and the supernatural are common. They often lack physical stamina. In appearance many are tall, thin and pale, and going grey or balding.

NOTES : The plant produces spore cases, on the end of upright forked stalks, and produces yellow spores and powder. Found in the northern hemisphere, native to moorlands, forests and mountains.

PART USED : Powder and spores.

BACKGROUND : Used as a remedy for digestive conditions and kidney disorders, as well as for treating gout.

Lycopus virginicus

Bugleweed; Virginia water; horehound; water bugle; gipsyweed

● Heart problems, including abnormalities of heart beat and palpitations, aneurysm, pericarditis, raised blood pressure, valvular disease, and heart failure. The sufferer may cough up blood.

● Goitre, a condition of the thyroid gland which results in a protrusion of the eyes.

Symptoms are exacerbated by physical exertion or exercise, excitement or agitation, and heat in any form. Things improve following sleep. but are also alleviated by pressure on the effected area.

NOTES : Plant with purple flowers and smooth, green leaves which give off an aromatic, minty odour. Native to North America.

PART USED : Whole fresh parts of flowering plant.

BACKGROUND : Used to treat bleeding in the lungs, as in tuberculosis, as well as heart conditions. The homoeopathic remedy was tested by the American homoeopath, Dr Edwin Moses Hale in the second half of the 19th century.

Lyssin

Hydrophobinum

● Severe disorders of the nervous system, including convulsions related to epilepsy, severe headaches, and preeclampsia. Preeclampsia (with fluid retention and high blood pressure) can lead to eclampsia, which is potentially life threatening and can produce convulsions, sometimes worse in the presence of running water.

● Anxiety associated with water and going mad.

People who are suitable often speak quickly, and are impatient and reckless, with an uncontrollable temper.

NOTES : Saliva of a dog which has rabies.

M

Magnesia muriaticum

Magnesium chloride

- Hepatitis with accompanying pressing pain in the liver when moving or when the area of the liver is touched. A feature is eating often which eases the discomfort in the stomach.
- Constipation where symptoms are exacerbated by salty food, being beside the seaside, and if having a bath. Stools are dry.
- Cramps, particularly in the thigh muscles.

Symptoms are worse when lying the right side, and from salt in any form.

Magnesia phosporicum

Magnesium phosphate

- Neuralgia, writer's cramp, spasms and cramp, which feature intermittent, shooting pains which can be brought on by a cold draught. They often predominantly effect the right-hand side.
- Colicky pains, such as gallstone colic and diverticulitis, which are relieved by bending over, and are alleviated by heat and firm pressure. Accompanying is a surfeit of wind but burping does not ease the symptoms. Irritable bowel syndrome and ulcerative colitis. Also colic in babies.

Symptoms are exacerbated by cold air and draughts,

by touching, at night, and when the sufferer is already fatigued and tired. Things are better with heat, and in warm surroundings.

People who are suitable tend to be academic and workaholics, and are sensitive, prone to worry, and thin in appearance.

NOTES : White compound obtained by reacting magnesium sulphate with sodium phosphate.

BACKGROUND : Essential for normal functioning of nerves and muscles, and a deficiency can lead to cramping pains and spasms, and is damaging to the heart and skeletal muscles. Schussler tissue salt.

Magnesia sulphurica

Epsom salts
● Warts. People who benefit tend to develop recurrent sore throats. There tongues are thickly coated and yellow in colour, but the edge and the tip are red.

Medorrhinum

Prepared from gonorrhoeal discharge
● Infection and inflammation of pelvic organs, menstrual pain, and pain in the ovaries. Also nappy rash.
● Some disorders of mucous membranes, the kidneys, and the spine, such as neuralgia.
● Asthma, especially when the sufferer feels better with their knees supporting the body and leaning on their elbows. Also angina with pain into the left arm and throat.

● Emotional disorders such as mood swings which feature change from extreme impatience and irritability to passivity. When impatient and irritable, the sufferer is always in a rush and may be selfish and insensitive. When withdrawn, the person is dreamy and forgetful, and feels at one with nature. The sufferer also feels – during both states – lost, deserted or neglected, and may also feel that everything is unreal as if they are in a dream. Also claustrophobia.

Symptoms are exacerbated by damp weather, over warmth in the early morning, during the day, and after urinating. Things are also worse with even slight movement, but things are better by lying on the front, during the evening, and when beside the sea. Symptoms are also alleviated by the sufferer resting on their hands and knees.

People who are suitable tend to have a family history of gonorrhoea and some forms of heart disease. They become anxious when anticipating forthcoming events.

NOTES : Gonorrhoea is a sexually transmissible disease, caused by the passing of a bacteria.

BACKGROUND : The disease has been identified since ancient times, and gonorrhoea can be passed from mother to baby during birth. It is potentially a devastating disease and is normally treated with antibiotics. Samuel Hahnemann believed that gonorrhoea was responsible for certain genetic traits or weaknesses in following generations. He called this a 'miasm', in this case the sycotic miasm. Two other miasms were identified: 'psora', identified with blisters and itching of scabies (*see* PSORINUM) and syphilis (*see* SYPHILINUM).

Mercurius corrosivus

Mercury chloride

- Severe symptoms of ulceration in the digestive and urinary tracts, and mouth and throat. These include ulcerative colitis, with severe diarrhoea containing both blood and mucus, and abdominal pains, as well as appendicitis.
- Severe bladder infections and urethritis with frequent, painful urinating, making the urine feel hot and scalding. Blood and mucus are present in the urine, as well as possibly a thick, discoloured discharge which contains pus.
- Ulcerated tonsils covered with a white, pus-filled discharge, facial pain, exhaustion, and secretion of excess saliva which tastes putrid. Gums may be swollen, and may also bleed, and the teeth may be loose.
- Congestive headache with a burning sensation in the cheeks.
- Depression where the sufferer loses all appetite, which is much worse during menstruation when the woman may feel suicidal. Also manic depression where the sufferer wants to flee and travel far away, and may have suicidal and homicidal thoughts.

Symptoms are worse in the evening, and when walking about, as well as by eating fatty meals and acidic foods. Things are better after eating breakfast, and with rest.

BACKGROUND : Highly poisonous, corrosive compound which results in burning and destruction of tissues if consumed.

Mercurius solubis

Mercury

● Conditions which produce a large amount of body excretions, which often smell unpleasant, can be yellowish-greenish in colour, and may contain blood. Accompanying symptoms can include burning up and heat, and intolerance to temperature.

● Fevers with profuse sweating.

● Inflammation of the gums, and bleeding or infected gums, gingivitis, swollen eyelids, bad breath, mouth ulcers, candidiasis, and excessive production of saliva. Also nappy rash, skin infections and varicose ulcers.

● Sore infected throats and colds with redness around the nose, especially where there is a greenish unpleasant smelling discharge, tonsillitis, mumps, infected ear with discharge, congested severe headaches, and pains in the joints. Nasal symptoms can be worse in warm conditions, and other features include a sore nose, bad breath, and periodic sweating which does not alleviate symptoms. Also pneumonia.

● Colicky pains, including the gallbladder.

● Parkinson's disease with weakness and trembling, stammering, and the need to flee.

● Also severe conjunctivitis, allergic conditions with a running nose, skin complaints which feature pustules, spots and ulcers.

Symptoms are exacerbated by extreme changes in temperature, draughts, and when the weather changes quickly, as well as by lying on the right side. Things are also worse when too warm in bed, at night, and if the sufferer sweats excessively. Things improve in a stable, comfortable temperature, and by resting.

People who are suitable can be prone to insecurity, although they can seem quite confident and calm on the outside. They tend to be cautious, introverted and aloof, and find criticism difficult as they become angry if disagreed with. They are excessively afraid of dying, going mad, thunderstorms, and burglary, and anxious about family members. They seem to always be hungry, and prefer bread, sugary food, butter, milk, and beer although they dislike other alcohol, meat, coffee, and salt. They can be fair-haired with fine, smooth skin.

NOTES : Metal which is liquid at room temperature.

BACKGROUND : Toxic, causing the production of copious amounts of saliva as well as vomiting, as well as many other problems. It was once used as a cure for syphilis.

Mezereum

Daphne mezereum; spurge olive; spurge laurel; flowering spurge; wild pepper; dwarf bay

● Tightness round the chest, persistent dry cough, and discharge of mucus from the nose.

● Halitosis which that smells of rotten cheese, with accompanying large production of saliva and the tongue tends to have a burning sensation which extends down into the stomach. There may well be a stomach ulcer.

● Impetigo with itchy and burning pustules which have red, inflamed skin surrounding them. They are worse when touched. Also psoriasis where white, thick crusts form on the skin, and shingles. After rubbing or scratching the rash or affected area the area feels cold. Also varicose ulcers.

Symptoms are worse in the cold, and also at night.

NOTES : Hardy shrub with dark-green leaves, purple-pink flowers, and red fruits. Native to Europe but also found in upland regions of North America.

PART USED : Bark.

BACKGROUND : Poisonous, but medicinal uses have been treating snake bites, toothache, and for helping ulcers. Causes redness and blisters if applied to the skin.

Moschus

Musk

● Hysterical, neurotic and emotional symptoms, which can include giddiness and fainting, palpitations, pallor and exhaustion, and sweating.

Things are made worse by resting, but also by moving about, during cold, fresh weather, and when excited or emotionally upset. Things improve after burping, and when in warm surroundings.

People who are suitable can be hypochondriacs, and may also believe that everyone is against them. They tend to talk a lot without pause, and have clumsy, hurried movements. They often feel cold, although only one side of the body feels chilled while the other is quite warm.

NOTES : Musk from the musk deer, a small deer found in hilly and mountainous parts of central Asia.

PART USED : Dried musk.

BACKGROUND : A strong odour secreted by the male musk deer to attract a mate. Used in perfumes from early times. Samuel Hahnemann was worried about the widespread use as he believed the substance weakened the immune system and made people susceptible to disease.

Murex
Purple mollusc
●   Menopausal symptoms of irregular bleeding.
●   Depression where the sufferer has emotional and hysterical symptoms, and may be anxious about their own health, particularly during menstruation.

    People who are suitable do not like being touched, and especially do not enjoy having to go through a medical examination.

PART USED : Body of the mollusc.

N

Naja tripudians

Cobra venom; naja tripudians

● Symptoms which predominate on the left side, especially of the heart but also of the left ovary. Symptoms present can include crushing, choking pain as in angina with pain extending down the left arm into the hand. Pulse may be slow, and breathlessness and choking can also feature. Also rheumatic heart disease.

● Asthma precipitated by hayfever.

Symptoms are exacerbated by lying on the left side, in cold draughts, and after sleeping, as well as by wearing tight clothes, and by drinking alcohol. Symptoms are also worse following menstruation.

PART USED : Dried venom.

BACKGROUND : Extremely poisonous, especially when sprayed into the eyes of its victims, causing blindness. Its bite can be fatal as it effects the heart and lungs, leading to collapse and death.

Naphthaline

Derivative of coal tar

● Hayfever and allergic rhinitis with accompanying sneezing attacks. Major features are red eyes and often a detached retina, and chest symptoms may develop into asthma. Also useful for cataracts and detached retina.

Symptoms are eased by being in the open air.

Natrum carbonicum

Sodium carbonate

● Eczema, chapped and dry sore skin, nettle rashes, cold sores, warts, moles, corns, blisters and other skin conditions.

● Sore throats, colds and conditions with catarrh, labyrinthitis, throbbing headache with nausea and vomiting, and indigestion, which can be brought on by draughts and where the nasal discharge is foul smelling. Symptoms can come and go on a daily basis, but are relieved by sweating. There may be a feeling of giddiness, as well as tinnitus and possible deafness. Symptoms can be worse premenstrually.

● Weak ankle which have a tendency to become sprained.

● Morning sickness with an associated craving for salt.

● Depression where the sufferer finds it hard to concentrate and to understand. Symptoms are worse during thundery weather.

Symptoms are worse in warm, humid weather and heat in any form, and may also be worse in noisy surroundings, but are alleviated by eating and by sweating.

People who are suitable tend to be warm, sensitive and intuitive, and are devoted to their friends and family. They can be positive and optimistic when ill, as much or more for others than for themselves. They are often delicate and have sensitive systems, tending to be intolerant of milk and dairy products, and can become quickly exhausted by physical activity. They are also very sensitive to music, and can get upset by noise and thunderstorms. Their ankles can be particularly weak, and are prone to strains and sprains.

BACKGROUND : Used medicinally for conditions such as creams and ointments for burns, eczema and other skin problems, as well as to help catarrh and vaginal discharge. The homoeopathic remedy was investigated by Samuel Hahnemann.

Natrum muriaticum

Salt; sodium chloride

● Conditions which arise from the functioning of the kidneys and the electrolyte balance of the body.

● Symptoms with production of a thin watery mucus, including colds and infections where there is a runny nose or other catarrhal problem.

● Some menstrual and vaginal conditions.

● Migraines and other headaches, candidiasis and ulcers of the mouth, cold sores with blisters on the sufferer's lips and chin, inflamed, bleeding and infected gums and gingivitis (the tongue is indented with teeth impressions). Also bad breath.

● Verrucas and warts, spots and boils, and cracked lips (often with a crack in the middle of the lower lip).

● Fluid retention such as urine retention, constipation with irregular bowel habit, anal fissure, indigestion, anaemia, and thyroid disorders. Also kidney disease when there has been exposure to malaria and quinine.

● Palpitations which make the body shake with

accompanying constriction around the chest.

● Cramps particularly in the legs, often with tingling in the lower limb.

● Suppressed grief and premenstrual tension, anxiety, tearfulness, depression, and over sensitivity and irritability.

Symptoms are exacerbated, or even brought on, by heat, either from the sun, a stuffy room or an open fire, although the sufferer may feel cold and shivery. Things are also worse during cold and thundery weather, in the late morning, in breezes by the sea, and by over exercising. The sympathy of others may also may make things worse. Symptoms are eased in the open air, sleeping on a firm mattress, and after sweating or fasting. A cold bath, swim or application can also help.

People who are suitable are often female, and are reliable and intelligent but prone to be serious and overly sensitive. They can take any criticism hard and deeply, and may have unrealistically high ideals. They desire the company of others but are easily hurt, and are afraid of losing control, insanity, and dying. Fear of failure, the dark, crowds, being burgled and claustrophobia can also be present. Music can move them to tears. In build they can often be squat or solid build with dark or fairish hair. They can be prone to red, watery eyes, as if they have been weeping, a puffy and shiny face, and cracked lips. They have a craving for salt, but do not like bread or fatty foods.

NOTES : Obtained from the evaporation of sea water or from rock salt.

BACKGROUND : Essential for many metabolic processes, including normal functioning of nerve tissues.

Natrum phosphoricum

Sodium phosphate

● Symptoms caused by an excessive amount of lactic or uric acid: excessive lactic acid can be caused by a diet too rich in dairy products and milk, as well as fatty foods. Other features include an excess of stomach acid, possibly because of eating too much sour food, as well as acid indigestion with a sour taste in the mouth, wind and abdominal pains. Excessive amounts of uric acid can are present in people suffering from gout with painful, inflamed, stiff joints.

● Depression where the sufferer is quite low, and may have auditory and visual hallucinations.

Symptoms are worse during thunderstorms, by consuming fatty, sweet or sour foods, and by physical exertion. Thing are better when out in the fresh clean air and in cool, airy surroundings.

People who are suitable can be somewhat timid, blushing easily, and can appear refined. They are quickly tired by any physical activity, but can be quite restless and appear agitated. They can be prone to depression and general dissatisfaction, but not readily accept advice.

NOTES : Obtained from a reaction between sodium carbonate and phosphoric acid.

BACKGROUND : Found in the body and involved in the regulation of acidity in body tissues and fluids, and in complex metabolic processes.

Natrum sulphuricum

Sodium sulphate

- Liver and gallbladder disorders including jaundice, digestive complaints with indigestion and colicky pains, severe chesty conditions such as bronchitis and asthma, and bladder problems with urinary frequency.
- Symptoms which arise after head injury, such as depression or personality change.

Symptoms are exacerbated by damp, cold conditions, by lying on the back, and are worse at night and during the morning at about 4.00 am. Things are better in cool, fresh and dry surroundings, for being out in fresh air, and symptoms are alleviated if the sufferer changes position.

People who are suitable can be excessively serious, and keep their feelings tightly controlled, hiding severe depression and thoughts of suicide. Their depression may be more apparent, and they can become quite emotional on hearing music or contemplating art. They can be a bit materialistic, and are very sensitive to damp weather with a tendency to suffer from asthma and chest conditions with catarrh.

BACKGROUND : Naturally occurring substance which is involved in metabolic processes. The compound was investigated by Schussler and is one of his tissue salts.

Nitric acidum

Nitric acid

- Sharp, stabbing splinter-like pains, often intermittent in nature, which are associated with piles or haemorrhoids, constipation, anal fissure, mouth ulcers and swollen salivary glands, warts, skin ulcers, severe sore throat with ulceration such as tonsillitis (feeling as if there is a fish bone in the throat), thrush infections, and ulcers in the stomach or duodenum.

●   Pneumonia with thick, yellow sputum, which can include specks of coagulated blood. Accompanying symptoms can be chapped, broken skin, often susceptible to warts or ulcers, which often feels cold. Urine or body secretions may have a strong pungent odour.

●   Kidney stones with renal colic which feels like the pain from splinters.

●   Depression where the sufferer is quite vindictive and irritable, and may have rages.

Symptoms are exacerbated by consuming acidic fruits and drinks, as well as milk, by touch or pressure, and by moving. They are also worse at night, but symptoms are alleviated with warmth, and in dry, warm conditions.

People who are suitable are often self-centred, egocentric and selfish, and can bear long-term grudges. They can feel that everyone is against them, and can fly into rages as they take offence too easily. They tend to be analytical, and examine events or perceived slights, and are often suspicious in nature. They enjoy salty and fatty foods when well. When they are ill, they are anxious that they might die.

NOTES : Obtained from a chemical reaction between sulphuric acid and sodium nitrate.

BACKGROUND : The concentrated acid is extremely corrosive. The acid has been used, after being very diluted, to treat severe infections and fevers, and to dissolve kidney or bladder stones. Externally to burn away warts.

Nux moschata

Nutmeg; Myristica fragrans

● Hysteria, agitation, excitement, exhaustion, drowsiness and confusion which follow an epileptic attack or stroke.

● Abdominal pain and indigestion, constipation, and inflammation of the gastrointestinal tract.

Symptoms are exacerbated by sudden changes in the weather, and damp and cool conditions. People who are suitable are often dehydrated and need to drink fluids, but they do not feel particularly thirsty. Symptoms are eased wearing warm clothing, for being warm, and during spells of high humidity.

NOTES : Tree with greyish-brown bark, dark-green, glossy leaves, small flowers, and red fruits when fresh. Native to southeast Asia but grown elsewhere.

PART USED : Inner seeds without husks.

BACKGROUND : In large doses causes drowsiness, giddiness and even fainting. Used medicinally from early times for digestive complaints and headache, and rheumatic pain. In herbal medicine it is used to sharpen eyesight.

Nux vomica

Poison nut; strychnos nux vomica; Quaker buttons

● Digestive complaints, such as indigestion, nausea,

vomiting, diarrhoea, constipation, cramps and colic. Also halitosis which smells of rotten cheese, piles or haemorrhoids with painful contractions of the rectum, and abdominal pains. Hepatitis with constrictive pains which extend to the right shoulder, and gallstone and kidney stone colic. Also colic in babies.

● Stomach complaints caused by overeating, especially rich food, coffee, drinking too much alcohol, and stress. Also associated palpitations. This is a useful as a hangover remedy, and for alcoholism.

● Migraines and other headaches, hayfever, allergic rhinitis, colds with redness around the nose and sore throat, dry coughs and flu-like symptoms of fever, aching muscles, chills and shivering, as well as irritability and teeth-grinding. These can have been brought on by cold and wet weather, or by draughts. The sufferer often feels cold, and the eyes are very sensitive to light.

● Cystisis and urinary frequency, as well as stress incontinence. Also urine retention following abuse of alcohol.

● Acne with blotchy skin which feels burning.

● Severe back pain, especially for women following labour. Other back problems.

● Heavy painful periods, morning sickness with a bloated abdomen, and labour pains.

● Epilepsy when the condition is brought on by being extremely angry.

● Impotence caused by too much work, alcohol or caffeine. The sufferer may also be a heavy smoker.

● Stroke brought on by over consumption of food or alcohol, or from overexertion or being soaked through.

● Mania where the sufferer is a workaholic and feels it

impossible to stop until things are perfect, even if it means working all hours.

● Night crying and insomnia by babies who wake up in the early hours and will not go back to sleep.

Symptoms can be worse in cold, windy and dry weather, in winter, after eating, and in the morning. Things are exacerbated by noises and music, bright light, touch, overwork, and eating spicy meals which cause nausea.

People who are suitable tend to be those in stressful jobs or who have stressful lives, and are ambitious and competitive, but can also be quite sedentary. They find it difficult to express their anxiety, although they can be passionate, and this leads to explosions of anger and excessive irritability. They also sometimes grind their teeth. Intolerance and the need for perfection also add to their tensions. They harbour excessive fears of dying and of failure, particularly in their work life, and do not like crowds. Many enjoy rich, spicy food, loaded with calories and cholesterol, as well as coffee and alcohol, although these foods can exacerbate their problems.

NOTES : Tree with grey bark, dark leaves, small pale flowers and orange (in colour), apple-like fruits with pale, hairy seeds. Native to parts of Asia, including India and the Malay archipelago.

PART USED : Cleaned and dried seeds.

BACKGROUND : Extremely poisonous as it contains strychnine. Used medicinally for various complaints including aiding digestion, cardiac function, and increasing urination. It was a cure for the plague in medieval times.

O

Ocymum canum
Bush basil

● Renal colic and stones which effect the right kidney, with the accompanying symptoms of pain, vomiting, cloudy urine with sediment, and urinary frequency. This may indicate an infection, and there can be a sharp pain on urinating, as in cystitis. The urine has a strong pungent smell of musk, and cramp-like pains affect the kidneys, mostly on the right side.

NOTES : Low, bushy plant which has a sweet odour. Native to parts of the Indian subcontinent.

PART USED : Fresh leaves.

BACKGROUND : Used medicinally for mild nervous disorders, and vomiting.

Oleander
Rose laurel

● Heart symptoms such as palpitations, weakness, extreme anxiety, and fainting. Accompanying symptoms may be giddiness or feeling on the point of collapse.

● Diarrhoea, nausea, sickness, abdominal pains, and other symptoms of gastroenteritis. Dry, chapped skin can also be present, as well as depression, lack of concentration, and clumsiness which can lead to falls and accidents.

● Vertigo, headache, blurred vision, muscular

weakness, and lack of co-ordination.

● Dermatitis and eczema.

Symptoms are exacerbated by undressing, walking, and are worse in warm conditions.

PART USED : Fresh leaves.

BACKGROUND : The remedy was investigated by Samuel Hahnemann

Opium

Opium poppy; papaver somniferum; mawseed

● Symptoms of mental shock as a result of a severe fright or emotional shock. Symptoms can either be of withdrawal and apathy, or alternatively of excitement, agitation and insomnia. Also present can be a greatly increased sense of hearing.

● Alcoholism with DTs, frightening hallucinations, and periods of unconsciousness following binges.

● Respiratory and breathing problems, constipation which can last for many weeks and is associated with a loss of appetite, as well as after a stroke.

● Urine retention which is painless but feels as if the bladder is about to burst.

● Stroke accompanied by paralysis with a feeling that the limbs have been severed.

● Epilepsy where the condition is brought on by being in conditions which are too hot.

Symptoms are exacerbated by sleeping, and in hot conditions, but are eased by moving and with exercise, and in cool surroundings.

NOTES : Plant with pale-pink flowers with a deeper

purple area at the base of the petals. Cultivated flowers come in a variety of colours. Native to Asia but cultivated in many other countries (often illegally).

PART USED : Unripened seed case.

BACKGROUND : A cut is made in the seed case and a milky white fluid, latex, is produced, which darkens as it dries: opium. Opium has various properties, not least as a narcotic, and is used in conventional medicine as a pain killer.

Ornithogalum umbrellatum

Star of Bethlehem; bath asparagus; dove's dung; star of Hungary

● Severe persistent digestive upsets, which feature burning pains, regurgitation of stomach acid, bloated abdomen, and flatulence. Also present may be peptic or duodenal ulcers, as well as depression and severe anxiety, irritability and short temperedness. There may be blood, either new or old like coffee grounds in any vomit, and burps smell foul.

NOTES : Bulbous plant with narrow, dark-green leaves, green and white flowers, and edible bulbs.

PART USED : Whole green part of the plant.

Oxalicum acidum

Sorrel acid; oxalic acid; common wood sorrel; Oxalis acetosella

● Painful rheumatic disorders, which predominantly effect the left side of the body. Pains are severe and sharp, and other features are weakness and feeling cold. There is a tendency for small haemorrhages called petechiae to occur, which show up as dark red spots beneath the skin. A tendency to bleed easily can also be present, and well as vomiting blood.

● Angina where there is a sharp pain in the left lung which can also be present in the left shoulder.

Symptoms are exacerbated by the sufferer thinking about themselves.

NOTES : Small plant with little, bell-shaped flowers veined with purple. Found in Europe.

PART USED : Leaves.

BACKGROUND : The leaves have a sharp and sour taste if eaten. Sorrel was used medicinally for fever, and conditions with catarrh, haemorrhages, and urinary conditions.

P

Paeonia

Peony

● Itchy piles or haemorrhoids, with discomfort and swelling.

● Sleep disturbance because of nightmares and indigestion, as well as feeling the need to sleep during the afternoon.

NOTES : Plant with deep pink flowers. Found in Europe, and often grown in gardens.

PART USED : Fresh root.

BACKGROUND : The plant was used in medicine from early times, and was believed to help prevent nightmares and epilepsy, convulsions and spasmodic nervous conditions, and was a cure for madness, and to help stop infection after giving birth.

Pareira brava

Ice vine; virgin vine; velvet leaf

● Urinary tract infections and conditions, such as cystitis, urethritis, urine retention and urine frequency. Hot burning pains may be present while urinating, as well as abdominal pain and discomfort. Also the pain from kidney stones.

NOTES : Vine with a twisted, knotted root. Native to parts of South America and the Caribbean.

PART USED : Root.

Paris quadrifolia

Paris; one berry; true love; herba Paris

● Conjunctivitis and inflamed, irritated eyes which are watery and itchy. The symptoms are worse on the left side, and the sufferer can be talkative and excitable.

NOTES : Herbaceous, perennial plant with whitish-green flowers which give off an unpleasant odour, and dark-purple fruit. Found throughout Europe and parts of Asia.

PART USED : Whole plant.

BACKGROUND : Poisonous and narcotic, causing vomiting, diarrhoea, giddiness, dry throat, sweating, and even convulsions and death. The remedy was investigated by Samuel Hahnemann.

Passiflora incarnata

Passionflower; maypops; passion vine; granadilla; maracoc

● Epilepsy or other conditions with convulsions or severe spasms, including whooping cough, asthmatic attacks, and tetanus.

● Mental conditions, with severe disturbance, such as DTs from alcoholism, and manic states.

NOTES : Perennial plant with perfumed flowers, which are flesh-coloured or yellow with tinges of purple, and large fruits, which are edible.

PART USED : Green parts of plant.

BACKGROUND : Used in medicinally for conditions such

as diarrhoea, dysentery, neuralgia, and insomnia.

Petroleum

Dry, cracked, chafed skin, particularly around the fingers, as well as chilblains and eczema. The condition is exacerbated in cold weather when the skin is heated then cooled.

● Sickness nausea and vomiting, especially where these are a result of travel sickness. Also present can be headaches, especially where these are focused on the back of the head.

● Halitosis where the breath smells of garlic. Accompanying symptoms include extreme hunger with a gnawing stomach ache when hungry. Sufferers may have to have to get out of bed in the middle of the night to get something to eat.

Symptoms are exacerbated by cold and windy weather, especially in the winter, as well as by thunderstorms. Things are better with warmth and warm dry weather, and after a meal.

People who are suitable may be prone to flying into rages, and can be hot-headed and excitable. Fatty foods upset them, and their sweat has a pungent odour. They often have inflamed, itchy sore skin, and this can be a reason for their irritation.

NOTES : Liquid crude oil.

BACKGROUND : Petroleum jelly is used for minor skin abrasions. The homoeopathic remedy was investigated by Samuel Hahnemann.

Petroselinum

Carum petroselinum; parsley; apium petroselinum;
petersylinge; persely; persele

● Cystisis where a feature is the agonising need to
urinate.

NOTES : Small green plant. Common.

BACKGROUND : Parsley is eaten, and is also used in herbal
medicine for gravel, stone, kidney congestion, dropsy,
and jaundice.

Phellandrium

Water dropwort; water fennel

● Chest and respiratory conditions, where symptoms
predominate on the right-hand side, and there is a sharp
pain in the right breast and breast bone. This can
include bronchitis and emphysema with breathlessness,
tuberculosis, a severe cough, and production of thick
mucus. Headache is also often present.

NOTES : Biennial plant with fruits which contain a yellow
fluid.

PART USED : Fluid from fruits.

BACKGROUND : In herbal medicine used to treat chesty
complaints such as bronchitis, asthma, intermittent fever,
and gastric conditions.

Phosphoricum acidum

Phosphoric acid

● Emotional and physical symptoms of exhaustion,
apathy, listlessness and depression, which may have been

caused by overwork or following a debilitating illness which has dehydration as a feature. Also present can be loss of appetite, feeling cold all the time, dizziness especially in the evening, and a feel of pressure pushing down on the head.

● Intestinal disorders with a distended abdomen and rumbling noises. Also present is diarrhoea, which cannot be controlled, along with a lot of flatulence.

● Growing pains in children, or who suffer from sleep disturbance.

Symptoms are worse in cold, damp, draughty conditions, and are exacerbated by loud noises. This improve after a good sleep, and in warm surroundings.

NOTES : Clear, crystalline substance.

BACKGROUND : Used in conventional medicine to treat tumours of the parathyroid gland as it acts on the blood and reduces levels of calcium. The homoeopathic remedy was investigated by Samuel Hahnemann.

Phosphorous

● Symptoms of acute anxiety, caused by stress and worry, and accompanied by exhaustion, insomnia, and indigestion. Symptoms are much worse during thundery weather.

● Gastric problems, including a burning sensation in the chest, gastrointestinal tract or abdomen, nausea and vomiting, diarrhoea, acid indigestion and heartburn, stomach ulcers, halitosis, and gastroenteritis. Sufferers are very thirsty and desire cold water. Also profuse diarrhoea with blood in the stools. The remedy helps those with bleeding duodenal or stomach ulcers. Nausea can be caused by exposure to tobacco smoke, and there are usually burning pains.

● Minor wounds, bleeding gums and gingivitis, nosebleeds and nasal polyps, and gastric and profuse menstrual bleeding.

● Respiratory conditions, particularly those with a severe cough and sore throat, accompanied by retching, vomiting, and also yellowish blood-tinged or rust-coloured phlegm, such as colds, laryngitis, bronchitis, tuberculosis, asthma, and pneumonia. There may also be crusts of dried phlegm. The sputum may have a considerable amount of blood.

● Conditions which include poor circulation and often recur, as well as varicose ulcers.

● Giddiness or labyrinthitis, especially in older people, experienced when moving from lying or sitting to standing.

● Cataracts and glaucoma where it feels as if a veil has been pulled over the eyes and coloured haloes appear around objects.

● Morning sickness with nausea and vomiting, which is worse in the evening.

● Night crying and insomnia in babies, even when they are neither hungry nor in pain.

Symptoms are worse in the morning and evening, and particularly before or during a thunderstorm. Over exercise, hot foods and drinks, and lying on the left side of the body can also make things worse. Symptoms are eased by being in the open air, by being touched, or stroked, after sleeping or catnapping, and when lying on the back or right-hand side. Gastric symptoms are eased by eating ice cream and cold food, although these can be vomited up once they have become warm in the stomach.

People who are suitable are often sociable and affectionate, and artistic and creative, and they improve when ill with company and sympathy. They need other people to fuel their optimism, and although they are usually positive, they may get little done. They are afraid of water, illness and dying, as well of the supernatural and the dark, and find thunderstorms particularly frightening. Most foods are enjoyed, but they can suffer from digestive problems. They are often attractive, tall and slim, and may have dark or fair hair.

BACKGROUND : Extremely poisonous. Medicinal uses included treating infectious diseases such as measles.

Physostigma

Calabar bean; physostigma venenosum; chop nut; ordeal bean

● Disorders in which there are muscle spasms, including conditions such as tetanus, meningitis, and poliomyelitis.

● Conditions which feature muscular and nerve degeneration, including multiple sclerosis, motor neurone disease, and Friedrich's ataxia.

● Diarrhoea, vomiting, fever, sweating, prostration, and palpitations, particularly when the pupils of the eye are contracted.

● Glaucoma, where the onset has been precipitated by trauma.

NOTES : Perennial, climbing plant with purple flowers which then produces pods with dark-brown seeds. Native of West Africa but now found elsewhere.

PART USED : Ripe seeds.

BACKGROUND : Seeds are extremely poisonous, and cause depression of the central nervous system, slowing of the pulse and a rise in blood pressure. Respiratory failure and death may follow. In herbal medicine used to treat eye problems, and it causes the pupil of the eye to dilate.

Phytolacca

Poke root; phytolacca decandragarget; reading plant; pocon; brenching grape; pigeon berry

● Hard lumps or tumours in the breast, either benign or malignant, as well as mastitis. The breast may feel hot, be swollen and painful to the touch, and stabbing pains can also be present.

● Severe sore throats, swallowing difficulty, and other conditions which features pain which can be referred to both ears, redness and inflammation, and feels as if there is a lump in the throat. Conditions include tonsillitis, pharyngitis and diphtheria. Also swollen salivary glands which are like hard lumps, often with sticky saliva.

Symptoms are exacerbated by swallowing, by movement, consuming hot drinks, and in cold damp draughty conditions. Things improve with warmth, and in sunny dry weather, by consuming cold drinks, and with having plenty of rest.

NOTES : Perennial plant with white flowers, clusters of shiny black berries, and an orange root. Native to North

America, but now also found in the Mediterranean, North Africa and China.

PART USED : Root.

BACKGROUND : Used by Native Americans to loosen the bowels, to cause vomiting, and as a heart stimulant, as well as for skin disorders. In Europe it was used for mastitis and breast lumps, and cancers. In herbal medicine used to treat skin disorders, ringworm and scabies, rheumatism, conjunctivitis, ulcers, and severe menstrual pain.

Pilocarpine muriaticum

Pilocarpine chloride

- Meniere's disease with tinnitus and deafness, but with profuse sweating as a feature.
- Swollen glands and mumps. The saliva is sticky.

Piricum acidum

Piric acid

- Extreme exhaustion which features apathy, indifference and severe fatigue, such as that experienced in post-viral fatigue syndrome and the syndrome commonly known as ME. It may be caused by bouts of intense intellectual activity such as studying for exams. Present is a general feeling of heaviness and lethargy, and the sufferer can be too tired to even conduct a conversation and cannot think clearly. Another feature is often a numbing headache with sore eyes, or there may be a boil in the outer part of the ear. This condition can also arise out of intense grief.

Symptoms are exacerbated by physical and intellectual activity, as well as being worse in hot surroundings. Things are better with rest and in cool conditions, and if the weather is sunny but not too hot.

NOTES : Obtained from a chemical reaction between nitric, sulphuric and carbolic acids.

BACKGROUND : Tested for homoeopathy in 1868.

Plantago major

Plantain; broad-leaved plantain; waybread; ripple grass
● Piles, toothache exacerbated by anything cold, and tooth abscesses and facial neuralgia
● Conditions such as diabetes where large quantities of urine are passed.

Symptoms tend to be on the left side, and are exacerbated by being in the cold, heat and draughts.

NOTES : Common plant with purplish-green flowers on spikes, and a rhizome. Found throughout Europe.

PART USED : Whole fresh plant.

BACKGROUND : Used medicinally since ancient times (and now in herbal medicine) to treat wounds and external bleeding, for venomous bites, and for disorders of the bowels and kidneys. Also as a remedy for piles or haemorrhoids, as well as diarrhoea.

Platina

Platinum
● Female sexual and reproductive conditions, with accompanying emotional problems. This can include

pain in the ovaries, spasms in vaginal muscles making it difficult to have sexual intercourse, heavy menstrual bleeding, absence or periods, and genital itching. Feelings of numbness may also feature, with chilling, muscle constriction, and the sufferer may have a dread of gynaecological examinations and procedures.

● Constipation where the stool is sticky, and there is a haste to defecate, but it seems impossible to perform an evacuation. The sufferer feels tall and everything looks small in comparison.

● Epilepsy with fits, but there is no loss of consciousness.

Symptoms are made worse by touching and physical contact, when tired, and in the evening, but improve when out in fresh, clean air.

People who are suitable tend to set themselves, and others, impossibly high standards, and may look down on other people. They often feel let down when they cannot match their own expectations, leading to depression and irritation. They believe that things were better in the past. This can lead to cynicism and contempt for others. They enjoy travelling to different countries.

NOTES : Precious metal.

Plumbum metallicum

Lead

● Long-term illnesses with sclerosis or hardening of the tissues as a feature, such as arteriosclerosis, atherosclerosis, multiple sclerosis, and Parkinson's disease.

- Colic, constipation with stools like small, hard balls, muscular weakness and tremor, and urine retention. There may be extreme pains.
- Stroke with paralysis, but pain in the affected area.
- Epilepsy where before the attack the legs feel heavy and go numb. Also present is a swollen tongue.

Symptoms are exacerbated by movement and are worse at night, while things are better with warmth and placing firm pressure or massaging the effected area.

People who are suitable have impaired concentration with their intellectual capacity dulled by sickness. A poor memory may be a feature as well as difficulty in expressing thoughts clearly. This can lead to the sufferer being lethargic and short-tempered.

NOTES : Metal.

BACKGROUND : Poisonous and can build up in the body, and particularly dangerous for children. Symptoms of poisoning can include persistent constipation, pale skin, a blue line along the gums and teeth because of lead sulphate, and muscle weakness. Intellect is also impaired and there are associated behavioural changes. Severe poisoning causes colicky abdominal pains, tremors, increasing muscular weakness and paralysis, and drooping wrists and feet. Convulsions and possibly death can follow.

Podophyllum peltatum

American mandrake; May apple; hog apple; wild lemon; racoonberry

- Vomiting and diarrhoea in gastroenteritis,

ulcerative colitis, gallstones, colicky pain, flatulence, and other digestive disorders. A feature may be bouts of alternating diarrhoea and constipation. The stools contain jelly-like mucus and smell very unpleasant.

Symptoms are worse first thing in the morning, as well as during hot weather, but improve by massaging the abdomen, and by lying on the front of the body.

NOTES : A herbaceous, perennial plant with large divided leaves and white flowers which have an unpleasant odour. The plant produces yellow fruits, which are edible, although the leaves and roots are poisonous. The roots and rhizome are yellowy brown in colour. Native to North America and found in wet meadows.

PART USED : Rhizome and roots.

BACKGROUND : Poisonous and causes nausea, vomiting and inflammation of the gastric tract, possibly leading to death. Used medicinally to treat deafness, liver and bowel complaints, dropsy, and to eliminate parasitic worms.

Polygonum

Smartweed; water pepper; biting persicaria; bity tongue; smartass; red knes; bloodwort

● Urticaria with small ulcers on the leg. Particularly useful for women going through the menopause.

NOTES : Annual plant with greenish-pink flowers and a black, dotted fruit. Native to Europe and parts of Asia.

BACKGROUND : Used medicinally for conditions such as gravel, colds and coughs, epilepsy, dysentery, gout, and bowel problems.

Primula veris

Cowslip; herb Peter; mayflower; key flower; key of heaven; fairy cups; pargle; peggle

● High blood pressure and the threat of a stroke with giddiness, confusion, headache, and the feeling that the heart is throbbing.

NOTES : Wild plant with yellow flowers. Found in Europe in woodlands.

PART USED : Flowers.

BACKGROUND : Used medicinally for conditions such as restlessness, headache, nervous debility, and insomnia.

Psorinum

● Conditions effecting the skin with dryness, cracking and soreness, and there may be infections with pus-filled blisters.

● Digestive problems, particularly featuring diarrhoea and indigestion, exhaustion, depression, and being gloomy in outlook.

● Hayfever, allergic rhinitis, asthma, general debility, irritable bowel syndrome, diverticulitis, as well as swollen eyelids, eczema, dermatitis, acne, boils and ulcers. Also bad breath with an ulcerated tongue and gums, which bleed easily.

● Depression where the sufferer feels that everything has gone badly and can see no hope for the future. They feel very cold.

Symptoms are worse in the cold, or when the weather turns cold, especially during winter weather, but also for being too hot: either while in bed, by strenuous exercising, or by wearing too many clothes. Things are better in the summer, in warm surroundings, and by resting with the arms and legs spread out.

People who are suitable are often gloomy in outlook, and fear that things are generally going to go badly. They are very sensitive to the cold, and may feel cold even during the height of the summer. They can experience gnawing hunger pains and headache, which is relieved by eating, and often they need to have a meal in the middle of the night. Their flatulence can smell of rotten eggs. They can feel family and friends have deserted them, and often believe that death is not far off.

NOTES : Derived from the fluid of scabies blisters.

BACKGROUND : Investigated by Samuel Hahnemann as he believed that the blisters produced in scabies were the result of a deeper illness. While the scabies blisters themselves might heal and disappear, this miasm (suppressed disease) would continue to cause disruption in the body, and might even be passed to following generations. Features associated with the scabies miasm are called psora.

Ptelea trifoliata

Water ash; swamp dogwood; wingseed; shrubby trefoil; wingseed; hop tree

● Hepatitis, liver enlargement and tenderness and other disorders, especially with discomfort and heaviness in the area of the liver.

● Indigestion and some other digestive conditions.

● Rheumatism.

Symptoms predominate in the right side of the body, and are worse when lying on the right side.

NOTES : Shrub. Native to North America.

PART USED : Bark of root.

BACKGROUND : Used medicinally for conditions such as debility, indigestion and poor digestion, and rheumatism.

Pulsatilla

Wind flower; pasque flower; meadow anemone; anemone pulsatilla

● Conditions where there is a greenish-yellowish discharge, such as colds and coughs, asthma, hayfever and allergic rhinitis, blepharitis and conjunctivitis, and sinusitis, earache and glue ear. The phlegm may be blood stained and smell unpleasant, and often the sufferer may have a lack of thirst. Symptoms may also be worse when in warm conditions, but come or go quickly, and there is a great variability in symptoms. Also for post-influenza weakness.

● Eye inflammations, as well as sties and conjunctivitis.

● Gastric complaints, particularly sickness, nausea, diarrhoea, heartburn, and indigestion caused by eating too much rich or fatty foods. Also haemorrhoids with accompanying pain.

● Palpitations caused by eating fatty food or by arguing.

● Osteoarthritis with pains which move about the joints. Also swollen tendons.

• Premenstrual, menstrual, and menopausal problems, as well as cystitis, particularly where these are accompanied by tearfulness, depression, and violent mood swings. Also morning sickness, particularly when brought on by smelling or eating fatty foods.

• Migraines and other headaches, epileptic conditions, rheumatic and arthritic conditions where there is inflammation and pain, and swollen glands, as well as nosebleeds. Also varicose veins, toothache, mumps, measles, acne, and chilblains.

• Cystisis and urinary incontinence, the latter which may be caused by coughing or passing wind. Also some prostate problems.

Symptoms are exacerbated by eating rich or heavy food, and when hot, during warm conditions, or being in warm room, and are worse at night. Things improve with light exercise and movement, and particularly when out in the open air, especially when it is cool and fresh. Crying can ease symptoms, as can the sympathy and care of others.

People who are suitable are often female, and tend to be gentle, loving and passive, but can be oversensitive and somewhat fastidious. They can be easily moved to tears, particularly by the suffering of others, both people and animals, although their tears may cause a sensation of 'burning'. They are usually sociable and popular, and prefer to avoid confrontation, but may find it difficult to be assertive. Fears can include being left on their own, illness, insanity, and dying, as well as the supernatural, the dark, and of crowds. Rich and sweet foods are often consumed, although they may upset digestion, and spicy foods are also enjoyed, although not fatty foods. They have a lack of thirst. In appearance they are usually attractive, although they can be a little overweight, and have blue eyes, smooth skin, and fair hair.

NOTES : Plant with purple flowers with orange middles. The flowers and leaves are covered in fine hairs. Native of northern and central Europe.

PART USED : Whole fresh plant is pulped and liquid extracted.

BACKGROUND : Used in medicine from medieval times for conditions such as whooping cough, asthma, bronchitis, leprosy, eye inflammations, and headaches.

Pyrogenium

Pyrogen: artificial sepsin

● Blood poisoning and other septic conditions where healing is slow. Accompanying symptoms are fever, aching bones, rapid pulse, sweating which does not cool the body, and feelings of heat and burning. The sufferer is uncomfortable and restless, even delirious, and there may be considerable pain from a septic conditions such as an abscess.

● Influenza where features include fever, restlessness, rapid pulse, cold and shivering, thumping heart, headache, and large frequency of urinating. With sore throats, a feeling that the mouth is full of pus may be a feature.

Symptoms are exacerbated by the cold and draughts, but are better for moving about.

BACKGROUND : Investigated by Dr John Drysdale towards the end of the 19th century. The remedy is derived from a mixture of raw beef and water which was left for three weeks, and after straining produced a liquid which was then mixed with glycerine. This substance, known as pyrogen, is believed to cause blood poisoning in large doses.

R

Radium

Radium bromide

- Eczema, moles, skin ulcers, acne, skin cancer, rosacea (a red, flushed face and enlargement of the skin's sebaceous glands), and dry, chafed, sore skin.
- Aching painful bones as in lumbago, rheumatism, and arthritic disorders, as well as bone cancer. Pain may move from one part of the body to another.
- Low blood pressure with accompanying weakness and palpitations on first waking.

Symptoms are worse at night, and when first moving after resting, but improve by lying down, or by moving about after a longer rest, and by having a hot bath.

NOTES : Compound of radium, a radioactive element.

BACKGROUND : Radium is used in radiotherapy for the treatment of cancers.

Ranunculus bulbosus

Buttercup; bulbous buttercup; crowfoot; St Anthony's turnip; gold cup; frogsfoot

- Shingles, eczema, and skin irritation and blistering, as well as rheumatism with hot, tearing pains.
- Pleurisy and bronchitis with accompanying pain during breathing. Other features are a feeling of being rundown and general malaise, bright-red cheeks, and a

clean tongue.

● Alcohol problems with trembling, irritability, headaches, and a crawling feeling on the top of the head.

Symptoms are worse during cold and damp conditions, and when the sufferer is afraid.

People who are suitable often have a problem with alcohol.

NOTES : Common, wild plant with yellow flowers and small swellings, which resemble tiny turnips, at the base of the stems. Found widely in Europe.

BACKGROUND : Contact with the plant can cause blistering and inflammation of the skin, and in herbal medicine it is used to alleviate the symptoms of gout, sciatica, and rheumatism, as well as helping headaches and shingles.

Ratanhia

● Rhatany; krameria triandra; krameria root; Peruvian rhatany.

● Constipation, anal fissure, piles or haemorrhoids, with extreme pain like broken glass in the rectum. Another feature is a feeling as if cold water is flowing over the molar teeth.

NOTES : Low-growing shrub with large, red flowers and strong roots. Native to Peru, where it is found in dry mountainous areas.

PART USED : Roots.

BACKGROUND : In herbal medicine used to treat diarrhoea, urinary incontinence, excessive menstrual bleeding, haemorrhage, and fissure.

Rhododendron

Yellow rhododendron; rhododendron chrysanthemum; snow rose; rosebay

●   Gout, rheumatism and arthritis with hot, painful swollen joints and severe tearing pain. Also osteoarthritis.

●   Neuralgic pains around the eyes and face, pain in the testicles, high fever with delirium and confusion, as well as severe headaches.

Symptoms are worse during the approach of a thunderstorm, at night, as well as being exacerbated by standing still for long periods, by resting, and at the onset of moving. Things are better following eating a meal, and improve with warmth.

People who are suitable are often quite anxious in nature.

NOTES : Low-growing bush with a reddish stem, oval leaves, and large, yellow flowers. Native to parts of Europe and Asia, where it is found in mountainous areas.

PART USED : Fresh leaves.

BACKGROUND : In herbal medicine used to treat rheumatic disorders, gout, and syphilis.

Rhus toxicodendron

American poison ivy; poison oak; poison vine

●   Inflammation of muscles, tendons and joints, and rheumatism, osteoarthritis, rheumatoid arthritis, sciatica, repetitive strain injuries, gout, lumbago, inflammation of the membrane round joints, as well as muscle stiffness, ligament and tendon strains.

● Eczema, acne, chilblains, cold sores, shingles, nettle rash and nappy rash, accompanied by burning feelings or dry and blistered skin.

● Fever-like symptoms of viral infections, including high temperatures, swollen, watery eyes, aching joints, pain throughout the body, nausea and vomiting, and shivering and chills. Conditions include colds, bronchitis, and influenza, especially where these are brought on by cold and wet weather.

● Back pain and lumbago which are alleviated by lying on a hard surface, by walking gently, and by bending over backwards.

● Parkinson's disease when the sufferer is very restless. Also present is twitching, trembling, stiffness, and cramps.

● Strokes, usually effecting the right side, which feels as if the effected area has gone to sleep.

● Depression where the sufferer feels anxious and despondent, and may think about drowning themselves. Symptoms are worse in the evening.

● Menstrual conditions, such as abdominal cramps and excessive bleeding, especially when these are relieved by lying down.

Symptoms are worse at night, by getting cold when undressing, following moving, and waking after a period of rest, as well as during stormy weather. Things improve when warm and dry, and by gentle movement or light exercise.

People who are suitable are often sociable, charming and entertaining, although they are prone to shyness when in new company. They work hard and take their work seriously, but can sometimes overdo it, and tend to exhibit some compulsive behaviour in order to function properly. They can get depressed, uneasy and anxious when ill, and are prone to tears.

NOTES : Small tree or large shrub which has off-white flowers and dun-coloured berries. Native to North America.

PART USED : Pulped leaves.

BACKGROUND : If touched causes an inflamed, painful and ulcerated rash. Other associated symptoms are headache, fatigue, malaise, fever, swollen glands and a loss of appetite. It was used medicinally to treat rheumatism, paralysis, arthritis, and skin conditions.

Robinia

Yellow locust

● Indigestion and heartburn, with acid and pain in the bowels. This remedy is suitable for children, especially when they smell sour.

Symptoms are worse at night, and when lying down.

Rumex crispus

Yellow dock; curled dock

● Skin conditions where itchiness is a major feature.
● Nasal congestion, and spasmodic coughs with latterly the production of copious amounts of thick, sticky mucus.
● Diarrhoea and digestive disorders.

Symptoms are exacerbated by the cold and draughts,

but improve with warmth and heat.

NOTES : Plant with large leaves which are curled and crisp at the edges. Common.

PART USED : Whole flowering plant.

BACKGROUND : Used in herbal medicine as a laxative and tonic.

Ruta graveolens

Rue; garden rue; herbygrass; herb of grace; bitter herb

- Bone, tendon, ligament, muscle and joint disorders, including sprains, bruising, fractures and dislocations, especially where there is a deep, tearing pain. Also synovitis, rheumatism, and sciatica.
- Respiratory problems such as painful deep coughs.
- Eyestrain due to tiredness and accompanying headaches.
- Infected or painful sockets following tooth extraction.
- Rectal conditions such as prolapse.
- Warts.

Symptoms are exacerbated in cold, damp conditions, after resting, lying down, and exercising out of doors. Things improve when warm or hot, and with light movement indoors.

When ill, those who are suitable exhibit anxiety, depression, and dissatisfaction.

NOTES : Hardy, evergreen plant with yellow-green flowers and an unpleasant smell. Native to southern Europe but grown elsewhere.

PART USED : Sap of green parts of plant, before flowering.

BACKGROUND : Poisonous, causing sickness, delirium and fits, and it should not be taken during pregnancy. Used in Chinese medicine for insect and snake bites, and other medicinal uses include to aid eyesight, as well as a remedy for coughs, croup, flatulence, hysteria, gouty and rheumatic pains, sciatica, and chilblains.

S

Sabadilla

Cevadilla; veratum sabadilla; asagracea offincinalis; cebadilla

- Symptoms of colds, hayfever and allergic rhinitis: spasmodic sneezing, running nose, watering itchy eyes which are red and swollen, coughing, headache above the eyes, and a sore throat.
- Elimination of threadworms.

Symptoms are exacerbated in the cold and in draughts, but improve in warm conditions, and while wearing warm clothes.

People who are suitable are usually nervous, timid, and can be easily startled.

NOTES : Plant which resembles a rush. Native to parts of North and Central America.

PART USED : Seeds.

BACKGROUND : Poisonous, causing severe vomiting and diarrhoea. Used medicinally to expel parasitic worms and lice, as well as to treat rheumatism, gout, and neuralgia. The plant produces symptoms similar to that of the cold: sneezing, running nose, watering itchy eyes, coughing, headache, and a sore throat.

Sabal serrulata

Sabal; sarenoa serrulata; sbala palm; saw palmetto;

palmetto scrub

● Enlargement of the prostate gland accompanied by slow difficult urinating with sharp pains. Sexual intercourse may also be painful, and also present are general fatigue and loss of libido. Also for inflammations of the testicles and breasts, where heat, swelling, and tenderness are present.

Symptoms are worse during cold, damp conditions, and when others are sympathetic, but improve with warm, dry weather and surroundings.

People who are suitable are often scared of falling asleep.

NOTES : Small tree, which resembles a palm, with a crown of large, serrated leaves and dark-brown, oval berries. Native to parts of the southern United States.

PART USED : Fresh berries and seeds.

BACKGROUND : Used in herbal medicine for tonic and sedative properties, including conditions with catarrh.

Sabina

Savine; sabina cacumina; savine tops; Juniperus sabina

● Rectal and uterine bleeding where burning or stabbing pains are a feature, as well as cystitis, heavy periods, and varicose veins.

● Gout and arthritic conditions with red, shiny swellings.

Symptoms are worse in hot conditions, but improve in cool, airy surroundings.

NOTES : Small, evergreen shrub with dark-green leaves and oval, purple berries. Found in parts of the Europe and the United States, although grown widely in gardens.

PART USED : Fresh spring growth.

BACKGROUND : Poisonous in large doses, and can cause uterine bleeding and abortion, gastric problems, and even death. Used in herbal medicine for skin conditions, such as warts, and to encourage the drawing out of infection.

Salicylicum acidum

Salicylic acid

● Giddiness where sufferers have a tendency to fall to their left-hand side, accompanied by headache and confusion when they try to stand up quickly.

● Tinnitus, with roaring and buzzing.

Salvia officinalis

Sage; garden sage

● Hoarseness and sore throats, mouth ulcers or ulcerated throat, and bleeding or infected gums, as well as wisdom tooth eruption or extraction.

Sanguinaria

Blood root; sanguinaria canadensis; red puccoon; sweet slumber; snakebite; coon root; Indian paint

● Chest and respiratory complaints, such as bronchitis, pneumonia, pharyngitis, asthma, rhinitis and polyps (small, fleshy projections) in the nose or throat. Accompanying symptoms include dryness and soreness, thirst, chest pain which extends to the right shoulder, profuse nasal discharge which is yellow in colour and smells unpleasant, and a croup-like cough. Also for whooping cough, colds and flu, hayfever, severe migraine, and similar throbbing headaches with visual disturbance, and rheumatic pains in the right shoulder.

● Acne with a blotchy rash around the nose, which burns and itches. Symptoms are worse in the spring.

● Hot flushes associated with hormonal levels in women. Also heavy periods also around the time of the menopause with sore nipples, especially the right one.

Symptoms often predominate on the right side, and are exacerbated by lying on that side of the body. Things are also made worse by touch and movement, and also worse be eating sweet foods, and during cold, damp weather. Things improve during the evening, following sleeping, and if the sufferer lies on their left side.

People who are suitable often appear red in the face, and their cheeks, soles of the feet and palms of the hands can have a periodic burning sensation.

NOTES : Perennial plant with white flowers and bulbous, fleshy roots with orange sap. Native to North America, where it grows in woodlands.

PART USED : Root, green parts of the plant, and seeds.

BACKGROUND : Poisonous in large doses, causing a burning sensation in the stomach with accompanying vomiting, thirst, giddiness, disturbed vision, and potentially collapse and death. In herbal medicine used for chest and respiratory complaints, such as bronchitis, pharyngitis, asthma, and polyps (small, fleshy projections) in the nose or throat.

Sarsaparilla

Smilax; red-bearded sarsaparilla; Jamaica sarsaparilla

● Bladder, kidney and urinary conditions, such as kidney stones causing renal colic, and cystitis. Also bladder stones. Accompanying features are frequent urination, although only small amounts may actually be produced, sharp burning pains, cloudy urine containing small deposits or stones, and some urinary incontinence, especially when sitting down.

● Rheumatism where the pains are worse at night, and during cold, damp and draughty conditions, especially in the spring.

● Eczema and dry skin with painful deep cracks and fissures.

Symptoms are worse at night, in cold, damp and draughty conditions, and skin conditions are worse in the spring. Things improve by standing, and uncovering the chest and neck.

People who are suitable often feel cold, and may have dry, scaly skin and spots.

NOTES : Plant with thorny stems. Native to Central and South America although now found in Europe and elsewhere.

PART USED : Fresh root.

BACKGROUND : Used as a treatment for syphilis, and smoke from the burning plant was believed to help asthma.

Secale comutum

Ergot; spurred eye

● Spasms in the arteries, such as in Raynaud's phenomena (numbness and blanching, redness and burning in the fingers and toes), cramp-like pain in leg muscles, uterine pains and contractions leading to bleeding irregularities, and ineffective contractions during labour. Also present is cold, numb skin but there are hot and burning feelings inside.

Symptoms are worse with heat in any form, or by being covered, but improve in cool, fresh air and conditions.

NOTES : Fungus found on various grasses such as wheat and rye grass. The spores of the fungus grow on the stigmas and at the top of the grass, and produce small black seeding bodies (sclerotia), which eventually fall of when the ears of the grass are ripe.

PART USED : The sclerotia are collected before the grass ears are ripe.

BACKGROUND : Poisonous if eaten with the cereal, and causes burning pains, a crawling feeling on the skin, delirium, convulsions, gangrene, collapse, and death. It also causes the uterus and smooth muscle to contract, and acts in the nervous system. In traditional medicine used to control post-partum haemorrhage following childbirth or abortion.

Sempervivum tectorum

Houseleek; Jupiter's eye; Thor's beard; jupiter's beard; bullock's eye

● Ulcers in the mouth and on the tongue, which bleed very easily, particularly at night. Also present can be a sore tongue with stabbing pains. The skin around the mouth can also have many blisters.

NOTES : Perennial, succulent plant with pale, red-purple flowers. Native to central and southern Europe but grown more widely.

BACKGROUND : Used medicinally for conditions such as burns and scalds, skin problems, warts and corns, and mouth ulcers.

Sepia

Ink of the cuttlefish

● Premenstrual tension, menstrual pain and heavy bleeding, infrequent or suppressed periods, symptoms brought about by the menopause, such as hot flushes, and postnatal depression. Also toothache during pregnancy, and particularly effective for early morning sickness, especially when nausea or sickness is caused by even the thought of eating.

● Conditions caused by imbalance of hormones, and where extreme fatigue and exhaustion are a feature, especially where there are muscular aches and pains. Also tuberculosis of the bones.

● Gastric problems, including sickness and nausea, abdominal cramps, wind and pain, when caused by eating dairy products, and headaches with nausea and giddiness.

● Cystisis, bladder stones, and incontinence.

● Hot and sweaty feet, veruccas, varicose veins, cold extremities, and other circulation disorders.

● Nettle rash, and urticaria.

● Back pain caused by a weak back. Symptoms are

relieved by pressing against something hard, and are exacerbated by kneeling or stooping.

● Depression where the sufferer withdraws and wants to be left alone.

Symptoms predominate on the left side, and are worse during cold weather, especially before a thunderstorm, in the late afternoon and evening, and early in the morning. Symptoms are also more extreme before menstruation, and when others are sympathetic. Things improve when warm or in hot conditions, and with quick, vigorous movements, keeping busy, and being outside in the fresh air.

People who are suitable are usually female, and seem aloof and self-contained, although somewhat inflexible and intolerant of others, especially when they disagree with them. They can be quick to anger, and bear grudges. They often enjoy going out and dancing, and can be successful but hard in their career – or alternatively feel they cannot cope, especially when looking after a family or home. Deep-seated insecurities are often harboured, and there is an extreme fear of being alone, illness, insanity, and loss of possessions and wealth. If ill, they like to be left alone and do not want sympathy. Often sour and sweet foods, and alcohol are enjoyed, but dairy products, bread and fatty meals can upset the system. In appearance they tend to be tall and thin, with a yellowish tinge to their skin, and some have a brown saddle-shaped mark on the bridge of their noses.

NOTES : The cuttlefish squirts out the ink when it feels threatened in order to hide its escape.

PART USED : Ink.

BACKGROUND : Used in medicine from early times. It was investigated by Samuel Hahnemann in 1834.

Silicea

Pure flint

- Disorders of the bones, nails and skin, and recurring infections and inflammations producing pus, where being rundown or having a diet deficiency is a feature.
- Colds, flu, tuberculosis, asthma, sinusitis, hayfever, allergic rhinitis, ear infections and glue ear and labyrinthitis. Nasal discharge can form hard crusts which cause bleeding when removed, and the tip of the nose is itchy. Another feature is sneezing attacks in the morning, and the sufferer is sensitive to light and the tear ducts swollen. Coughing can become violent when the sufferer lies down.
- Boils, warts and carbuncles, skin abscesses and varicose ulcers, sties and cataracts, and varicose ulcers and infections of the fingernail.
- Gingivitis and gum infections where the gums are sensitive to cold air.
- Conditions of the nervous system, such as epilepsy. Also overwork and insomnia caused by overwork, and some headaches.
- Aiding the body expel splinters in the skin and other foreign bodies, also useful for expelling tooth fragments after an extraction.
- Constipation when it is difficult to complete evacuation of the stool with accompanying colicky pain.
- Bladder stones.

● Anxiety and phobias associated with pointed objects, such as pins and needles.

Symptoms are exacerbated when in cold and wet conditions, draughts, when swimming or bathing, by becoming cold when undressing – and are worse on the left side. Things are improved in the summer, when warm or in hot surroundings, by wearing warm clothing, especially a hat or other head covering, and by not lying on the left side of the body.

People who are suitable are often self-effacing and lacking in confidence, and they often get extremely fatigued from even gentle exercise. They are usually hard-working and diligent, sometimes overly so, and are neat and tidy to the point of obsessiveness. They can be unassertive and feel they are put upon by others, and they fear failure and dislike exercise as it exhausts them. Cold food and drinks are enjoyed. They often have sweaty, smelly feet and are afraid of needles. In appearance, they are thin with a light build, with pale skin and fine, straight hair.

NOTES : Mineral commonly founds in rocks and sand.

PART USED : Ground flint.

Solidago virgaurea

Woundwort; golden rod; solidago; Aaron's rod

● Urine retention, inability to urinate, and renal colic.

● Prickly heat with an itchy rash, which is mainly on the lower limbs.

NOTES : Plant with yellow flowers. Found in Europe, Asia and North America.

PART USED : Green parts of plant.

BACKGROUND : Used from early times for kidney and urinary conditions, particularly kidney stones.

Spigelia

Pinkroot; spigelia anthelmia; annual worm grass

● Symptoms which predominate on the left-hand side, especially heart disorders and palpitations, which may be violent with accompanying breathlessness and sharp pain which extend into the arms. This includes angina and coronary artery disease with severe, stitching pain. The sufferer may also have halitosis, and desire hot drinks which can relieve the pain. Also rheumatic heart disease.

● Neuralgia, left-sided throbbing headache and migraine, and iritis, which all feature sharp pains.

Symptoms are exacerbated by lying on the left side, in cold surroundings, by touch and by moving, and during the approach of a thunderstorm. Things are better in warm and dry conditions, by lying on the right side with head held high, nd during the evening.

People who are suitable tend to have a phobia about needles and other sharp, pointed objects.

NOTES : Perennial plant which has an unpleasant odour. Found in parts of South America and the Caribbean.

PART USED : Dried plant.

BACKGROUND : Poisonous in large doses. It was used to expel parasitic worms.

Spongia tosta

Natural sponge

● Thyroid gland conditions and goitre, where features are palpitations, sweating, flushing, breathlessness, heat intolerance, anxiety and nervousness. Also disorders of the pancreas which have the same symptoms.

● Heart disorders, such as an left-sided heart failure, enlarged heart or valvular disease. Symptoms include palpitations, pain, breathlessness and wheezing, exhaustion and a crushing sensation. Also present can be flushing, anxiety, and fear of death.

● Hoarse, dry, sore throat and laryngitis, especially where there is a family history of respiratory diseases such as tuberculosis. Croup, especially when breathing sounds like a saw being cut through a board.

Symptoms are exacerbated by movement, touch, by lying with the head low, trying to talk, by consuming cold drinks and meals, in cold surroundings, but improve with warmth and warm meals and drinks, and by sitting in a propped-up position.

People who are suitable are often light haired and skinned, and are thin in appearance.

PART USED : Roasted sponge.

BACKGROUND : Used in medicine from early times to treat goitre, enlargement of the thyroid gland caused by a deficiency in iodine, either from a metabolic problem or because of a lack of dietary iodine. Sponges are rich in iodine.

Stannum metallicum

Tin

● Severe chest complaints with thick, yellowish catarrh and a hoarse, dry cough as main features, such as asthma, bronchitis, larnygitis, and inflammation of the windpipe. Also present can be weakness and debilitation, weight loss and exhaustion, accompanied by depression and weepiness.

● Neuralgic pain and headache, particularly where this predominates on the left side. There may be a gradual onset of the pain, which can also be slow to disappear.

● Cramps, contractions and weakness which effect the hands.

Symptoms are exacerbated by lying on the right side, and consuming warm drinks, but things improve for coughing up catarrh, and putting firm pressure on the painful area.

NOTES : Soft, silver-coloured metal.

BACKGROUND : Poisonous in large doses, and used medicinally from early times to eliminate tapeworms.

Staphysagria

Lousewort; delphinium staphisagria; stavesacre; staphisagris; planted larkspur

● Neuralgic pain, toothache, pain from surgical operations, and pressure headaches.

● Gingivitis with loose teeth which are black and crumbling, toothache, as well as bad breath and bleeding gums. Also teething in children.

● Recurrent sties, especially where the eyeball is

surrounded by blue rings and are hot. Also present are itchy and sometimes swollen eyelids.

● Cystisis with urine frequency and pain, and useful when undergoing surgery of the urinary tract. Disorders of the prostate gland. Also can reduce pain during sexual intercourse for women.

● Warts.

● Stiff joints and repetitive strain injuries.

Symptoms are exacerbated by suppressing emotions, following a sleep in the afternoon, and after breakfast. Things improve with warmth, and by giving vent to pent-up feelings.

People who are suitable often appear to be quite relaxed and mild on the outside, but inside they can be a seething mass of emotions, especially anger and irritation. They can bear grudges against those they believe have insulted them, and may be workaholics. They can be afraid of losing control, but often have a high sexual drive. Their body excretions may smell unpleasant, and they particularly enjoy sweet foods and drinking alcohol.

NOTES : Large, annual plant with hairy stems and leaves, spikes of light blue or purple flowers, and pods containing dark seeds. Native to southern Europe and parts of Asia, although now found more widely.

PART USED : Seeds.

BACKGROUND : Extremely poisonous, and even in small doses acts as a purgative, causing diarrhoea and vomiting. Used since early times to kill parasites including lice, and as an external application to treat scrofula, skin eruptions, as well as insect bites and stings.

Sticta

Lungwort; sticta pulmonaria; oak lungs; lung moss

● Colds, asthma, lung inflammation, and rheumatic disorders, particularly when a feature is that catarrh is difficult to cough up and when it is persistent.

● Joint pain in the knee with swelling, tenderness and spasmodic pain. Also swollen tendons with shooting pains.

Symptoms are worse at night, in cold, damp surroundings and when lying down, but improve in warm conditions.

NOTES : Plant with oval leaves dotted with white spots. It produces flowers, which are red at first but deepen to purple as the flower matures. Found in Europe where the plant is widely grown in gardens.

PART USED : Whole fresh plant.

BACKGROUND : Used in herbal medicine for coughs, lung conditions, and asthma, as well as reducing inflammation and pain.

Stramonium

Stramonium; datura stramonium; thornapple; devil's apple; stinkweed; devil's trumpet; map apple

● Nervous system disorders, especially in children, including spasms and twitches, muscular jerking, convulsions, high fever in children, and meningitis and strokes. Also epilepsy where fits are triggered by bright lights or dancing images, and headaches which cause the sufferer to become incoherent while their vision is blurred. Also alcoholism with DTs.

● Symptoms of receiving a severe shock, night terrors in children, chronic anxiety, mania and agitation. Depression where the sufferer swings between excitement and despair. They sufferer may be violent, both verbally and physically.

● Urine retention which is eased by drinking vinegar.

Symptoms are worse following sleeping, in the dark, when the sufferer is alone, if the weather is overcast, and when the sufferer tries to swallow food. Things improve with reassurance and company, and in light and airy surroundings.

People who are suitable often have irrational fears: children may have night terrors, while adults are unduly terrified of violence or water. They can be quite loud in behaviour. There is often a need for orange or lemon juice, or other acidic drinks, and an excessive thirst.

NOTES : Large, bushy plant with white flowers then large capsules, protected by thorns, containing dark seeds. The plant has an unpleasant odour except for the flowers. Found throughout most temperate areas of the world.

PART USED : Juice from green parts just before the plant flowers.

BACKGROUND : A narcotic, and poisonous in larger doses. It was used from early times to help asthma, rheumatism, sciatica, haemorrhoids, abscesses and boils, and other inflammations.

Streptococcin

Streptococcol bacteria

● Kidney disease following acute tonsillitis.

Strontium carbonate

● High blood pressure with accompanying generalised pains which are centred in the bone marrow.

Sulphur

Flowers of sulphur; brimstone

● Dermatitis, eczema, psoriasis, and a dry and flaky, itchy skin or scalp. Also nappy rash.

● Gastric conditions such as reflux, and indigestion caused by an intolerance to milk or dairy products.

● Haemorrhoids, intermittent constipation with large hard stools, and diarrhoea worse in the early morning.

● Premenstrual and menopausal problems such as hot flushes.

● Conjunctivitis and eye inflammations.

● Lower back pain

● Colds with redness around the nose, and coughs with catarrh when associated with draughts, pleurisy, migraine headaches, and symptoms associated with fevers. The sufferer often sweats easily and gets overheated, and many conditions have stitching pains.

● Asthma.

● Crampy pains in the calf muscle, particularly the left.

● Symptoms associated with stress and worry, such as insomnia, irritability, fatigue, and lethargy, and depression where the sufferer cries for no reason.

● Impotence where the sufferer consumes a lot of fatty foods and alcohol.

Symptoms are usually worse around 11.00 in the morning, and in stuffy, hot and airless conditions.

Symptoms are also exacerbated by being too hot in bed or during the day, by washing or taking a bath, and by standing or sitting for a long time. Things are also worse when drinking alcohol. Symptoms improve in dry and warm surroundings, by taking light exercise, and by lying on the right side.

People who are suitable can appear somewhat dishevelled and untidy, and have dry, flaky skin and coarse hair. They may be thin or overweight, and tend to slouch and to be round-shouldered, as well as to have a round and rather red face. They can be lively, warm and intelligent, but somewhat impractical and fussy, and they need to be praised. They enjoy a wide range of food, often showing a preference for fatty foods, and they like alcohol, but can exhibit an intolerance to milk and eggs. Fear of failure in work, of heights, and of the supernatural can also be present, and they can suffer from frightening dreams. They often feel hungry around 11.00 am, and have hot feet at night.

NOTES : A yellow powder which when burnt smells like rotten eggs.

BACKGROUND : Used since early times in the belief that it could ward off infectious diseases because of the foul smell. It is found in body tissues, and in traditional medicine is used to treat some skin diseases.

Sulphur iodatum
Sulphur iodide
● Acne with persistent pustules erupting in the face. The face is always red, and sufferers feel as if their hair is standing on end.

Sulphuric acid

● Mental exhaustion and depression, especially where agitation and restlessness are present. Skin problems may also be a feature, such as ulcers and boils, mouth ulcers, and bleeding gums, as well as depression.

● Crampy conditions of the hands with fingers that jerk.

Sumbul-perula

Musk root ferula sumbul; euryangium

● Left-sided heart failure, often with nervous and hysterical symptoms, palpitations, and a persistent pain around the left side of the breast.

● High blood pressure with accompanying palpitations in a nervous individual whose blood pressure rises by just thinking about it.

NOTES : Tall plant with large leaves. Native to Russia and parts of Asia.

BACKGROUND : Used medicinally for hysteria as well as menstruation problems.

Symphytum

Comfrey; symphytum officinale; knitbone; knitback; blackwort; bruise wort; boneset

● Helps broken and fractured bones and blunt penetrating injuries to heal, including injuries to the eye.

NOTES : Plant with drooping creamy-yellow or purple flowers. Native to Europe and parts of Asia.

PART USED : Root and leaves.

BACKGROUND : Used medicinally for intestinal troubles, diarrhoea and dysentery, whooping cough, and haemorrhages. Externally it was (and is) used for cuts, sprains, swellings and bruising, and for soothing pain.

Syphilinum

Syphilis

● Chronic ulcers and abscesses, especially in the genital area.

● Menstrual pain, neuralgia, varicose veins, constipation, and iritis. Other features can be pain in the long bones, and weak teeth.

● Angina with pain behind the breastbone.

● Asthma.

● Phobias and anxiety.

Symptoms are exacerbated by great heat or cold, are particularly bad during the night and when lying down, when near the sea, and during a thunderstorm. Things improve by taking gentle exercise or walking, during the day, and when in a mountainous area.

People who are suitable tend to be somewhat nervous and anxious, and may have a nervous tic or muscular twitch. Obsessive behaviour may be a feature, such as continual washing of hands or checking that a cooker is switched off. Concentration and memory may be poor, and there may also be a problem with alcohol, other drugs, and smoking.

NOTES : Bacterial material obtained from a syphilitic lesion. A nosode.

BACKGROUND : Syphilis is a sexually transmitted disease,

and is passed by a bacteria. Samuel Hahnemann believed that syphilis was one of the miasms, which could lead to inherited problems in later generations.

T

Tabacum

Tobacco

- Nausea and vomiting, such as travel sickness, vertigo and disorders of the organs of balance found in the ears. Nausea is brought on by the slightest movement.
- Pain from kidney stones, along with a cold sweat and nausea, and a feeling of burning heat in the abdomen.

Symptoms are exacerbated by even slight movements of the head, in hot conditions, and from tobacco smoke, but things improve after vomiting, and in cool surroundings.

NOTES : Plant with hairy stem and leaves. Native to America, although now cultivated in many parts of the world.

PART USED : Fresh leaves of the plant.

BACKGROUND : Used by the native peoples of South America, but was brought to Europe in the 16th century, and is the main constituent of cigarettes. The plant contains nicotine, which is poisonous and causes sickness and nausea, palpitations, sweating, headache, and giddiness. It has been established that smoking is a major cause of premature death, although tobacco has been used medicinally for hernias, constipation, tetanus, worms, and hysterical convulsions.

Tarantula cubensis

Cuban tarantula

● Abscess, boils, carbuncles, infections of the fingernail, as well as genital itching, especially where these recur.

● Shock and anthrax, and can be used for severe conditions as a last resort. The infected areas can often be tinged blue, and pain, often burning, is most severe at night.

● Urine retention where it is not possible to relax their bladder spincter. Commonly with gastrointestinal upset.

Symptoms can be exacerbated by physical exercise, by drinking cold drinks. Symptoms are eased by smoking tobacco.

NOTES : Venom.

BACKGROUND : Poisonous, but does not appear to work right away. After about a day the area of the bite becomes inflamed and red, to be followed by swelling, fever, and an abscess.

Tarantula hispania

Spanish spider

● Jerking limbs in sufferers who find it impossible to stay still. Also epilepsy when the sufferer becomes unconscious without warning, as well as multiple sclerosis.

● Cystisis with accompanying high temperature and gastric symptoms.

People who are suitable tend to be very sensitive to the needs of others, but are extremely restless, hurried and fidgety. They find music relaxes them.

Taxus baccata
Yew
● Skin infections with blisters and accompanying night sweats where the perspiration smells extremely unpleasant.

NOTES : Large tree with red-brown bark, dark, glossy leaves, and fruits which can be red or yellow. Found in Europe, north Africa and west Africa.

BACKGROUND : Extremely poisonous, but a preparation of the leaves was once used to treat epilepsy. The tree can live for hundreds of years, and is often grown in churchyards.

Tellurium
Tellurium
● Bad breath where their is a smell of garlic, with an accompanying craving for apples.
● Sciatica which predominates on the right side.

Symptoms are exacerbated by straining to defecate, as well as by coughing and laughing. Other back problems.

Terebinthina
Turpentine
● Infections involving inflammation and infection of the bladder and kidneys, including cystitis with frequent urinating, blood in the urine and burning pains, and

kidney infections with stabbing back pains. The urine is often cloudy or contains blood, and it may have a strong odour like violets.

● Other forms of kidney disease with symptoms of fluid retention such as puffiness. Also urine retention with accompanying spasms whenever the sufferer attempts to urinate, as well as cutting, burning pains in the bladder. It may be associated with a sexually transmitted disease.

Symptoms are worse at night, as well as in cold, damp and draughty conditions, but improve for walking about in fresh, clean air, as well as in warm conditions.

NOTES : An oily, aromatic resin, which is obtained from some coniferous trees.

BACKGROUND : Causes burning if consumed with vomiting and diarrhoea. It can also cause external burning and blistering, and choking, sneezing and coughing if the fumes are breathed in. It was formerly used in the treatment of genital infections, such as gonorrhoea.

Teurcrium marum

Cat thyme; teurcrium marum venum

● Polyps, which may be found in the rectum, bladder or nasal passages, which can cause irritation and itching.

● Conditions where thick catarrh is a feature, especially when this is persistent and difficult to eliminate, with accompanying sneezing, and the production of nasal discharge.

● Threadworm in children.

Symptoms are exacerbated during cold and damp conditions and sudden weather changes, and are worse in the evening, and after becoming hot and sweaty in bed. Things are better when out in cool, fresh and clean air.

NOTES : Shrub with small, furred oval leaves and pink flowers. Native to Spain but found more widely.

PART USED : Fresh parts of the plant.

BACKGROUND : Used in herbal medicine.

Theidion

Orange spider

● Conditions sensitive to movement, vibration and noise which cause great pain. These include Meniere's disease, a condition of the inner ear with deafness and tinnitus, which also features vertigo, nausea and vomiting.

● Low blood pressure where the pulse rate is usually slow and with giddiness. Pain radiates from the heart to the left arm and shoulder.

● Toothache, degeneration of bone and spine with inflammation and pain, morning sickness, travel sickness, vertigo, severe headache, chills, and fainting.

● Tuberculosis.

Symptoms are exacerbated by closing the eyes, by any kind of movement or vibration, as well as by bending, touch, and are worse during the night. Things improve by resting with open eyes, by being in warm conditions, and in quiet and peaceful surroundings.

Those who are suitable can be overly sensitive, even

hypersensitive, and shrill sounds penetrate into their teeth. They become nauseous with motion, which is much worse when the eyes are closed.

NOTES : Small spider covered with orange spots. Native to parts of the Caribbean

PART USED : Whole spider.

BACKGROUND : Poisonous bite causes tremor, chilling, sweating, fainting, and extreme anxiety. The remedy was tested by Dr Constantine Hering in the 1830s.

Thuja occidentalis

Arbor vitae; yellow ceda; arbor vitae; tree of life; American arbor vitae

● Warts, fungal infections, and wart-like tumours on any part of the body. Also nasal polyps.

● Shingles.

● Asthma, often following a recent immunisation, with sweating on uncovered parts of the body

● Some conditions of the genital and urinary tracts, such as cystitis, urethritis, and prostate problems.

● Pain on ovulation and other inflammations and infections.

● Infections of the mouth, teeth and gums, conditions with thick green catarrh which may contain blood and pus, and for tension headaches.

● In-growing toe nails with ridged and brittle nails.

Symptoms are worse during the night at around 3.00 am, in the afternoon, after eating in the morning, and after being too hot in bed. Symptoms are also worse when the weather is cold, damp or wet. Things improve with movement and light exercise, massage, and after sweating.

People who are suitable tend to sweat profusely, a condition which can be helped by this remedy. They can suffer from insomnia, and during periods of sleep they may talk or cry out. Dreams can be troubled, including falling from a height. Often they can wake with an intense left-sided frontal headache. They are often insecure, try to please others, and are very sensitive to criticism, often becoming depressed. In appearance they can be pale and thin, dishevelled or untidy, and may have greasy skin.

NOTES : A coniferous tree with leaves which have a strong aromatic smell like camphor. North America.

PART USED : Fresh green leaves and twigs.

BACKGROUND : Used for a wide variety of ailments, including coughs, fevers, gout, dropsy, scurvy, rheumatism, warts, and fungal infections. It can induce abortion. A preparation is used in aromatherapy.

Thyroidinum

Thyroid gland of a sheep

● Psoriasis which is associated with obesity. The sufferer's hands and feet are generally cold.

Tuberculinum

Tuberculinum

● Chronic conditions which feature wasting, pallor, a persistent dry racking cough, drenching sweats at night, and pains in the left lung. Also present are enlarged glands in the neck, and the whites of the eyes may appear slightly blue. Symptoms are also erratic and may move about the body. There may be a family history of tuberculosis or another severe respiratory condition such as asthma. Conditions include colds with dried catarrh and yellowish nasal discharges, which are worse while in warm surroundings.

● Asthma or angina with palpitations and heaviness about the heart, where there is a family history of tuberculosis

● Crohn's disease, with early morning diarrhoea. The stools smell extremely unpleasant and are produced explosively.

● Anxiety and phobias associated with dogs and other animals.

People who are suitable have a personal or family history of tuberculosis. They tend to be restless and seek constant change in their personal lives. Often they need excitement which is provided by travel and new relationships. They are prone to being afraid of cats and dogs, but enjoy milk and the taste of smoked foods. They lack physical strength and stamina, and may be prone to colds and chesty complaints. In appearance they are often fair haired, blue eyed, and tend to be thin.

NOTES : Dead and sterile tuberculosis tissue, a nucleo-protein, derived from cattle or humans.

BACKGROUND : Investigated by Dr Compton Burnett in the late 1800s, following an earlier discovery, by Dr Robert Koch, that dead tuberculosis material was effective in the prevention and treatment of tuberculosis.

U

Urtica urens

Nettle; common nettle; stinging nettle

●   Conditions which cause burning and stinging of the skin, including nettle rash itself, insect bites and stings, skin lesions caused by burns and scalds, and eczema.

●   Nerve inflammation and pain, shingles, rheumatism, gout, and cystitis, especially where there are burning stinging pains.

Symptoms are exacerbated by touch, and are worse in cold, wet or snowy weather, and with contact by water. Things improve if the affected skin is gently rubbed, and if the sufferer lies down and rests.

People who are suitable are usually prone to skin conditions featuring inflammation, itching and irritated skin, and can be restless, impatient and fretful.

NOTES : Common plant. Hairs on the leaves produce a skin irritant when brushed, causing painful white bumps to appear. Found widely in Europe, Asia, Japan, South Africa and Australia.

PART USED : Fresh green parts of the plant.

BACKGROUND : Used from early times to treat conditions such as asthma and bronchitis, rheumatism and muscular fatigue, consumption or ague, and to ease insomnia. The new leaves can also be eaten, or brewed into tea and drunk.

Uva ursi

Bearberry; rchostaphylos uva-ursi

● Bladder stones where the urine flow has been stopped. Urine is ropy and thick with mucous sediment. It burns the sufferer.

● Kidney disease.

NOTES : Trailing, evergreen and woody plant with shiny leaves, white flowers, and bright, red berries. Native to Europe, Asia and America.

BACKGROUND : Used in herbal medicine for conditions such as urethritis and cystitis.

V

Valerian officinalis

Great wild valerian; all-heal; setwall; capon's tail

● Agitation, restlessness, and anxiety.

● Conditions with muscular spasms, hysteria, headache, and pains which may move about the body. Other features are insomnia, diarrhoea, and restlessness with gnawing hunger and nausea.

NOTES : Plant with dark leaves, pink flowers, and a rhizome. Found throughout Europe and parts of Asia.

PART USED : Rhizome.

BACKGROUND : Used medicinally since early times for conditions such as debility, insomnia, epilepsy, to prevent cholera, and to strengthen eyesight.

Veratum album

White hellebore

● Severe conditions of shock and collapse, which feature pallor, dehydration, chilling, and possibly a blue tinge to the skin caused by a lack of oxygen. Skin may be cold and clammy.

● Low blood pressure with an irregular pulse, as well as conditions with an irregular heart beat.

● Diarrhoea.

● Intense throbbing headaches.

● Severe depression where the sufferer feels impending doom and waits in a stupor. Also agitation, as well as suicidal impulses, mania and aggression.

- Cholera.
- Severe menstrual pain with cramps, cramp during pregnancy which can lead to fainting.
- Collapse because of mental shock or trauma.
- Bronchitis with coldness and weakness, and where a rattling chest is a feature. Also pneumonia.

Symptoms are exacerbated by moving, by consuming cold drinks, and are worse during the night. Coughing can be exacerbated by moving from a warm room to a cold area. Things improve with warmth and heat, consuming hot food and drinks, by resting, and by lying down.

People who are suitable tend to be somewhat aggressive and quarrelsome, and they may have a red, angry face.

NOTES : Plant with white flowers and a rhizome. Found in many parts of Europe.

PART USED : Rhizome.

BACKGROUND : Extremely poisonous, causing diarrhoea, vomiting, collapse, convulsions, and death. Used for medicinal purposes from early times, and in homoeopathy investigated by Samuel Hahnemann in the 1820s.

Viola tricolour

Wild pansy; love-lies-bleeding; love-in-idleness; heartease

- Infected eczema, impetigo, and skin conditions where thick pus-containing discharge, and crusts and scabs on the skin, are a feature.

● Urinary incontinence and bed-wetting.

NOTES : Plant with rounded leaves and coloured flowers, which can be purple, yellow or white. Common.

PART USED : Whole plant.

BACKGROUND : Used medicinally from early times for asthma, epilepsy, convulsions, skin conditions, and heart and blood disorders. Also used in herbal medicine.

Vipera

German viper

● Phlebitis and varicose veins and ulcers, where swelling, inflammation and pain are a feature. Also present may be a heavy feeling in the leg as if it might burst.

Symptoms are made worse by touching or applying pressure, and by wearing tight clothing, but are alleviated by raising the effected area.

NOTES : Poisonous snake, grey in colour, with a dark chevron pattern down its back.

PART USED : Venom.

BACKGROUND : The bite of the adder, which is painful but only occasionally serious, causes swelling, inflammation and bleeding in the veins, which then become enlarged.

Viscum album

Mistletoe

● Last resort remedy to treat extreme conditions of collapse, weak pulse and respiration, and low blood pressure.

● Sciatica, with shooting, tearing pains in the limbs, gout or rheumatic conditions.

NOTES : Parasitic plant which lives on oak, fruit and other trees, and has white berries. Found throughout Europe.

PART USED : Leaves and twigs.

BACKGROUND : Poisonous. Used in herbal medicine for epilepsy, spasms, and haemorrhage.

Z

Zincum metallicum

Zinc

● Agitation, restlessness and nervous spasms or twitching. A feature is excessive mental and physical exhaustion, and also present can be irritation, sensitivity to noise, touch or interruption. Also epilepsy where the condition occurs during another illness.

● Depression where the sufferer may cry when they are furious, but they fear that they are going to be punished for a supposed crime.

Symptoms are exacerbated by the suppression of discharges (by using a suppressant remedy in the case of a cold), as well as by noise, touch, vibration, and alcoholic drinks, especially wine. Things improve when natural body functions are allowed to proceed normally.

NOTES : Metal.

BACKGROUND : Essential for normal health, and is part of digestive enzymes. Used in conventional medicine as a constituent of skin creams and ointments. It is also taken internally for some nervous conditions, spasms and neuralgia.

allergic rhinitis irritation of the mucous membrane of the nose by allergens such as grass and tree pollen and fungal spores. Symptoms are stuffiness, nasal discharge, and sneezing.

aneurysm weakness in a blood vessel wall, causing swelling, which may burst, resulting in a haemorrhage and severe problems if this is in an important vessel in the brain or aorta.

angina central constricting chest pains, caused by the heart muscle not getting enough oxygen. It may herald a heart attack.

appendicitis inflammation of the appendix, which is potentially life threatening, with pain in the lower right part of the abdomen which is worse when the area is touched.

arthritis inflammation of the joints or spine, with swelling, pain, redness, heat and warmth of the skin, and restriction of movement. It can be caused by osteoarthritis, rheumatoid arthritis, infective arthritis, and tuberculosis.

asthma narrowing of the airways in the lung which causes distressing and potentially life-threatening breathing difficulties. It normally appears in childhood, and is caused by a sensitive response to allergens present in the environment, as well as stress, exercise and infection. Also present may by eczema and hay fever.

atherosclerosis build up of cholesterol on the walls of the arteries which results in a reduced blood supply to the heart muscle.

atrophy wasting of part of the body due to ageing, lack of use, malnutrition or illness.

barotrauma condition of the ears, with pain and temporary deafness, caused by sudden changes in pressure, such as experienced in an aeroplane.

blepharitis inflammation of the eye lid.

boil an infection of a gland or hair follicle with inflammation and pus.

bronchitis inflammation of the upper airways in the lungs which can be caused by infections. Accompanying symptoms include coughing, wheezing, chest pain and pain on coughing, and pus-containing mucus. If the condition spreads into the bronchioles it can lead to lack of oxygen. Bronchitis can be fatal and is a common killer among the elderly, particularly in those who smoke, live in damp housing or in a cold and damp climate, and who suffer from other respiratory infections.

bruises injured tissue can leak blood even if there is no open wound, and this area appears discoloured, going from black and blue to brown and yellow as the injury heals.

burns burns are caused by dry heat, electrical current and chemicals, and can cause serious damage to tissues. If burns are deep, the tissue may not be able to regenerate.

cancer tumours and growths which can invade surrounding tissues and disrupt or destroy them. Cancerous cells can be spread through the system, either via the blood or lymphatic system, and form secondary tumours or growths. Common causes of cancer include smoking, nuclear radiation, ultraviolet (sun) light, viral infections, and the presence of cancerous genes.

candida infection by candida albicans, which can effect the mouth, throat, vagina, skin and stomach. It can cause conditions such as thrush and pulmonary disease.

carbuncle inflamed and infected hair follicles and the

surrounding tissue.

carcinoma cancer.

cataracts condition where sight starts to become misty, and the lens of the eye can become cloudy and opaque, with possible blindness.

chilblain itchy, round inflammation of the skin which is usually caused by cold weather and a deficiency in circulation of the blood.

cholera infection of the small intestine by a bacteria, which can vary from relatively mild cases of vomiting and diarrhoea to severe cases of dehydration and death. Epidemics of cholera which occur in overcrowded conditions with poor sanitation can kill up to 50% of those effected.

colic severe pain which is caused by a spasm in one of the organs of the abdomen, such as the intestine or uterus.

cirrhosis liver disease, which can be caused by alcohol abuse or viral hepatitis, although this is not always the case. Liver tissue is damaged and dies, which can prove fatal.

conjunctivitis inflammation of the membrane of the inside of the eyelid and front of the eye, with redness and swelling, and the eyes are very watery.

constipation condition when the sufferer does not or is not able to pass faeces, which become dry, hard, and difficult and painful to pass. Regularity of bowel and bowel habit varies greatly between individuals. Attention to diet, eating more roughage and taking exercise can increase bowel frequency, as can laxatives and enemas. Some life-threatening conditions can cause constipation, including tumours, and is can also be present in other conditions.

consumption tuberculosis of the lungs.

convulsions rapid muscular contractions, spasms and relaxations in the limbs and body, which are caused by brain disturbance as in epilepsy, extreme fever and meningitis.

cramp prolonged, painful muscular contractions which usually occur in the limbs but can also occur is some of the internal organs. It can be caused by a salt deficiency because of heavy sweating. Other cramps, such as writer's cramp, are caused by excessive and repetitive use of an action using the same muscles.

Crohn's disease condition of the bowel where the colon wall becomes thickened and chronically inflamed, and possibly ulcerated. Symptoms are abdominal pain, diarrhoea, weight loss, and it can lead to a serious blockage of the intestine.

croup condition which features a partial obstruction to the larynx, usually in young children, making breathing difficult with a crowing sound, and sometimes accompanied by coughing and fever. Diphtheria is one cause of the condition, and very occasionally croup can be life threatening.

cyanosis lack of oxygen in body tissues which leaves the skin with a bluish tinge.

cystitis Inflammation of the bladder, usually caused by a bacterial infections, which is more common in women. Symptoms can include painful urination and frequent need to urinate, fever, and blood in the urine.

delirium state with confusion, agitation, anxiety, fear, illusions, and sometimes hallucinations, which can be caused by fever, poisoning, stress, shock or poor nutrition.

depression condition which features gloominess, sadness and even deep despair, along with other potential symptoms such as loss of libido and appetite, sleep disturbances, lack of energy, hopelessness, and suicidal feelings.

dermatitis types of eczema

diarrhoea increased frequency and looseness of bowel movement which involves the passing of very soft or liquid faeces. The condition is usually caused by food poisoning, along with irritable bowel syndrome, colitis, dysentery among many others. Severe diarrhoea can be dangerous because of loss of salts and fluid, particularly in the very young.

diphtheria serious, infectious disease which can cause respiratory and gastric problems, and even damage the heart and nervous system. The disease, which is caused by a bacteria, is commonest among children and can be fatal, although it is possible to immunised against the disease.

diverticulitis infection of small pouches in the wall of the colon, with localised, persistent pain, and possible vomiting and fever. Symptoms can be similar to the early stages of cancer.

dropsy old term for oedema or fluid retention.

dysentery infectious disease which involves ulceration of the lower bowel, causing severe diarrhoea with mucus and blood. There is more than one form of the disease, but it is spread via infected food, water or by contact with an already infected individual. Accompanying symptoms can include indigestion, nausea, anaemia, weight loss, cramp, and fever.

eclampsia a severe manifestation of toxaemia in pregnancy, with symptoms of convulsions, fits and coma.

eczema inflammation of skin with a red rash and possibly blisters which weep and become encrusted. The rash is also extremely itchy. There are several different kinds of the conditions, although it is usually caused by allergies or stress.

endocarditis inflammation of the inner lining of the heart, usually because of rheumatic disease.

epilepsy a neurological condition which involves seizures, convulsions and usually loss of consciousness. It can be caused by trauma to the head, brain tumours, cerebral haemorrhage and metabolic problems such as hypoglycaemia. An attack can often happen without warning.

erysipelas skin condition, caused by a bacteria, with inflammation and redness. Also present can be fever, pain, and a feeling of heat as well as tingling.

fistula an abnormal opening in the body, which may occur between organs or glands and the exterior. These can be caused by various factors including injury, **infection**, following surgery, or a baby may be born with the condition.

flatulence wind or gas with gastrointestinal tract distension.

Friedrich's ataxia Progressive childhood disease where the sensory and motor areas are effected, causing muscular weakness and staggering.

gallstones stones which form in the gallbladder and can cause severe pain and also obstruct the bile duct and cause jaundice. They appear to be caused by cholesterol stopping being soluble, and contain a proportion of **calcium** salts, and may form around a foreign body.

gastroenteritis condition where the stomach and intestine become inflamed, with symptoms such as diarrhoea and possibly vomiting. The cause is usually a virus. Dehydration is a problem, especially in children.

gingivitis infection of the gums which can cause the gums to deteriorate and the teeth become loose and possibly fall out.

goitre enlargement of the thyroid gland, with symptoms such as nervousness, weight loss, and palpitations.

glaucoma condition where the pressure inside the eyeball is increased, possibly causing severe pain and blindness. Symptoms include red eyes and the cornea appearing cloudy.

gonorrhoea common sexually transmissible disease which is usually spread via sexual intercourse. Symptoms include pain on urinating with a discharge of pus, and possible inflammation of organs such as the testicles and prostate in men, and the uterus and ovaries in women. If left untreated the disease can lead to arthritis, heart problems and conjunctivitis. It is possible for a mother to pass the disease to her baby during childbirth.

gout condition caused by an excess of uric acid which leads to inflammation of effected joints, arthritis and destruction of the joint. The kidney may also be damaged with the formation of stones. Deposits can reach the stage where they prevent further movement of the joints and they end up set in one position.

gravel small stones which can form in the urinary tract, which are formed from calcium salts and crystalline matter. Expulsion of the stones from the kidney usually causes great discomfort and pain, and there may also be blood in the urine.

haemorrhoids also known as piles. Inflammation of veins and varicose veins located at the end of the bowel in the wall of the anus. They are usually caused by constipation or persistent diarrhoea, especially in middle and older age, and may be exacerbated by a sedentary lifestyle. Pregnant women also commonly get haemorrhoids. Symptoms can include bleeding and pain.

hayfever an allergic reaction to allergens in the air, such as grass pollen and fungal spores. Symptoms include nasal discharge, sneezing, watery eyes, and itchiness. Hayfever can lead to asthma, and eczema may also be present.

hysteria condition which features a range of symptoms including seizures, paralysis and spasms of limbs, mental disorders and amnesia. It can be caused by emotional excitement, although the condition itself is difficult to define.

impetigo infectious disease, caused by a bacteria, where rashes with blisters are normally found around the nose and mouth. The condition usually effects children, and the rash is highly infectious.

influenza highly infectious viral disease which affects the respiratory tract and includes headache, weakness, fever, aches and pains, and loss of appetite. It can also be responsible for serious lung infections. The disease can be fatal, and the elderly or those with heart conditions are particularly vulnerable. The illness is sometimes mixed up with colds, but influenza is a much more serious condition.

insomnia sleeplessness.

iritis inflammation of the coloured part of the eye, which can lead to blindness.

jaundice liver condition which leads to bile pigment in the blood which makes the skin look yellow, as well as the whites of the eyes. There can be various causes, including obstructive where the bile does not reach the intestine because of a gallstone, red blood cells being destroyed by haemolysis, and liver disease such as hepatitis.

labyrinthitis infection of the middle ear which controls balance. Symptoms include giddiness which may cause falling down, and possibly nausea and vomiting.

laryngitis inflammation of the lining of the larynx and vocal cords, which is usually due to a viral infection, although there can be other causes including overuse of the voice, heavy smoking, chemical irritants and bacteria. It can also accompany infections of the upper respiratory tract such as colds and include coughs, difficulty in swallowing and pain.

lumbago condition of the spine, where the sufferer is unable to move, with accompanying back pain.

malaria infectious disease which is caused by a parasitic organism transmitted to man by mosquitoes. The disease features recurrent bouts of fever and anaemia, shivering and sweating.

mastitis inflammation of the breast.

Meniere's disease condition with symptoms of giddiness and deafness. Giddiness may cause nausea and vomiting, and deafness may be associated with tinnitus.

migraine condition with a throbbing headache, with symptoms such as an aura with flashing lights, nausea and vomiting, and temporary paralysis or pins and needles in a limb or even lip. The sufferer normally feels exhausted after an attack.

motor neurone disease disease with degeneration of the nerves which control muscle. Symptoms are atrophy of muscles, twitches, and later difficulty walking and swallowing.

multiple sclerosis Progressive disease which effects the nerves, although there can be periods of remission.

Symptoms include pins and needles in the limbs, urgency and frequency of urination, one hands which does not work properly, and a painful eye.

mumps an acute infection of the parotid glands, which is situated in front of and below the ear, caused by a virus.

nephritis inflammation of the kidney, which can be caused by infection.

neuralgia nerve pain, which includes sciatica, pain affecting the face and intercostal pain in the chest, which can have a variety of causes.

oedema fluid retention within the human body, which can be quite localised due to injury or effect the whole body which can be caused by heart or kidney failure. Fluid can collect in the chest cavity, abdomen or lungs (when it is called pulmonary oedema). Oedema can have many causes including cirrhosis of the liver, heart and kidney failure, acute nephritis, allergies, drugs and starvation. Women can also suffer from oedema during menstruation, which manifests itself as swollen legs or ankles.

osteoarthritis aching joints and other joint problems caused by wear and tear on the joint, and there is commonly pain on movement. It is usually a problem in the elderly, but may be caused by injury.

osteosclerosis increased density and hardness of bone.

palpitations the rapid and forceful beating of the heart, of which the sufferer is aware.

palsy paralysis, although the term is now only used for certain specific conditions such as cerebral palsy.

pleurisy inflammation of the pleura, which results in pain from deep breathing and breathlessness. Often associated with pneumonia, or disease of the lung, diaphragm, chest wall or abdomen, including conditions such as tuberculosis, abscesses or bronchial carcinoma.

Parkinson's disease condition with symptoms which include tremor in the limbs, shuffling gait, blank expression, muscular rigidity, and also a pill-rolling movement in the fingers. The disease can be degenerative, and also present can be depression or dementia..

pericarditis inflammation of the outer membrane of the heart.

pharyngitis inflammation of the pharynx, a cavity at the back of the mouth

phlebitis condition where the wall of a varicose vein becomes inflamed.

photophobia condition where there is an intolerance to light with accompanying pain. It can be symptoms of several illnesses, including viral infections, influenza and ME-type conditions.

pleurisy inflammation of the lining of the lung, which can be caused by an infection. Symptoms are severe pain whenever the sufferer breathes in.

pneumonia infection of the lungs, caused by bacteria, viruses or a fungus, resulting in inflammation and the filling of the lungs with pus and fluid. The lungs is starved of oxygen, and symptoms include chest pain, coughing, breathlessness, fever and possibly cyanosis, where the skin get a blue tinge from lack of oxygen.

poliomyelitis polio virus which can cause paralysis.

prolapse when an organ or tissue moves from its normal place in the body because the supporting tissues have weakened. This can occur in the vagina or uterus because of injury during childbirth.

psoriasis skin disease, which has no known cause, which

features scaly, itchy skin, which is red. The disease normally begins around the elbows and knees. There may be a genetic element, and the conditions is associated with anxiety.

Raynauld's phenomenon condition where the fingers and also possibly the toes become numb, white or bluish and stiff. It is caused by poor circulation, and as circulation returns to normal the digits are effected by pins and needles.

rheumatism general term to describe pain in the joints and muscles.

rosacea skin disease with red flushed areas, especially in women during the menopause.

scarlet fever infectious disease, which normally strikes in childhood, and is caused by a bacteria. Symptoms include sore throat, sickness, fever and a possibly widespread red rash.

sciatica pain in the sciatic nerve which is felt in the back of the thigh, leg and foot. It often caused by a prolapsed disc in the spine.

sinusitis inflammation of the sinus of the nose and head, with symptoms such as a blocked nose, pain, and possibly fever.

smallpox highly infectious disease, which is caused by a virus, and the symptoms of which are a fever, vomiting, and headaches and pain in other parts of the body. Red spots appear on the skin which then eventually become pus filled and which leave scars. The sufferer remains infectious until all the scabs are gone. The fever can return with delirium. The disease had been all but eradicated, and the last case was reported in 1977.

synovitis inflammation of the synovial membrane, which

lines parts of joints.

syphilis an infectious, sexually transmitted disease which is caused by a bacteria. Symptoms, in the first stage, are an ulcer and then the hardening of lymph nodes throughout the body. Some two months or so later secondary symptoms occur with fever, pains, enlarged lymph nodes and a faint rash usually on the chest. The final, tertiary stage may not emerge for up to many years and consists of numerous tumour-like growths throughout the body which can cause damage to the heart, brain or spinal cord causing blindness, mental disability and tabes dorsalis. Syphilis can be transmitted across the placenta from the pregnant woman to her unborn child.

thrush infection by a yeasty, fungal infection, with symptoms such as itchiness, redness, and a milky discharge. The infection can be passed by sexual contact, although it may also be caught spontaneously.

tinnitus a persistent ringing, buzzing or humming in the ears, which can be caused by ear wax, some drugs and by damage to the ears by noises which are too loud.

tuberculosis several infections which are caused by a bacteria of which pulmonary tuberculosis of the lungs is the best known. The pulmonary disease, which can be carried without symptoms, may lay dormant for years, but severe symptoms include fever, wasting, night sweats, and coughing up blood. The disease can also be contracted through contaminated food and many effects the abdominal lymph nodes leading to peritonitis. The disease is usually vaccinated against in developed countries.

ulcer a cavity in the skin surface or mucous membrane which may become inflamed and fail to heal. This can include bedsores and varicose ulcers, which are caused by defective circulation, as well as duodenal ulcers, gastric ulcers and peptic ulcers.

ulcerative colitis ulceration of the colon with pain, painless diarrhoea which may contain blood and mucous. It can lead to cancer of the colon if it persists for many years.

urethritis inflammation of the passage from the bladder through which urine passes. Symptoms include a discharge of pus from the penis and just behind the clitoris, with accompanying pain, itchiness, alteration in bladder habit, and possibly also a fever.

urticaria rash, much like nettle rash, with raised weals, swelling and itchiness. The conditions is usually caused by an allergy to shellfish or other foods, to some drugs, as well as stress and exposure to certain plants such as nettles and poison ivy.

varicose veins veins which become stretched, distended and twisted. Superficial veins in the leg are often effected although it may occur elsewhere. Causes can include obesity, pregnancy, inflammation of the wall of a vein with secondary thrombosis, and congenital defective valves.

verucca kinds of wart, including that commonly caught by children on their feet, although they can appear on other parts of the body. They can be highly contagious.

whitlow nail-bed infection.

whooping cough infectious disease caused by a bacteria and which affects the mucous membranes of the air passages. Symptoms are fever, catarrh and a characteristic cough, which features a number of short coughs punctuated with a 'whooping' drawing in of breath. Nosebleeds and vomiting may also be present. The illness can be dangerous in children and young infants, and they can be immunised.